Practice Issues
in HIV/AIDS Services
*Empowerment-Based Models
and Program Applications*

Practice Issues in HIV/AIDS Services

Empowerment-Based Models and Program Applications

Ronald J. Mancoske, DSW
James Donald Smith, ACSW
Editors

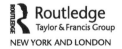

Routledge
Taylor & Francis Group

NEW YORK AND LONDON

First Published by

The Haworth Press, Inc., 10 Alice Street, Binghamton, NY 13904-1580.

Transferred to Digital Printing 2009 by Routledge
270 Madison Ave, New York NY 10016
2 Park Square, Milton Park, Abingdon, Oxon, OX14 4RN

Cover design by Marylouise E. Doyle.

Library of Congress Cataloging-in-Publication Data

Practice issues in HIV/AIDS services : empowerment-based models and program applications / Ronald J. Mancoske, James Donald Smith, editors.
    p. cm.
Includes bibliographical references and index.
ISBN 0-7890-2301-6 (Case : alk. paper) — ISBN 0-7890-2302-4 (Soft : alk. paper)
    1. HIV-positive persons—Services for. 2. AIDS (Disease)—Patients—Services for. I. Mancoske, Ronald J. II. Smith, James Donald.

RA643.8.P73 2003
362.196'9792—dc22

2003021010

In Memoriam

CONTENTS

ABOUT THE EDITORS

Ronald J. Mancoske, MSW, MPA, LCSW, DSW, is Professor of Social Work and Chair of the Health/Mental Health curriculum at Southern University in New Orleans. He has volunteer experience with various HIV/AIDS services programs (research centers, primary care centers, hospices, housing programs, emergency care sites, counseling programs), and is prior chair of the Ryan White Planning Council. He has published numerous book chapters and journals on HIV/AIDS services and is author of *Empowerment Practice, Rural Social Services for Gay Men and Lesbian Women,* and co-author of *Rural Gays and Lesbians: Building on the Strengths of Communities.* His current research and practice interests are in the intersection of poverty and deprivation, and their impacts on health and mental health programs and services.

James Donald Smith, ACSW, GSW, is Associate Professor and Director of Student Affairs in the School of Social Work at Southern University in New Orleans. He has more than 20 years of experience working with persons with HIV/AIDS individually and in groups. He is past Chair of the HIV/AIDS NASW Committee in both Mississippi and Louisiana. Among other publications, he is co-author of *Rural Gays and Lesbians: Building on the Strengths of Communities.* His primary interest in research is focused on HIV/AIDS and human service programs.

CONTRIBUTORS

Karen Davis is completing a dual master's program in social work and public health at Boston University. In 1999, she received her bachelor's in anthropology and psychology from the University of Texas at Austin. She is currently a research coordinator at the Center on Work and Family at Boston University.

Faith Ferguson, PhD, received her doctorate in sociology from Brandeis University. Dr. Ferguson is currently a senior research associate at the Center on Work and Family at Boston University, where she has worked on analysis of the data from the current three-year study. She has an extensive research background, including work as a research analyst in management consulting, where the focus of the work was race and gender issues in the corporate workforce.

Therese Fitzgerald, MSW, is a research associate at the Center on Work and Family at Boston University's School of Social Work. She received her master's degree in clinical social work at Boston University. She is currently pursuing a doctorate in social work and sociology at Boston University. Her research interests include the substance abuse treatment needs of mothers and women of color. She can be reached at the Center on Work and Family, Boston University School of Social Work, Boston, Massachusetts, e-mail: <tfitzger@bu.edu>.

DeAnn Gruber, LCSW, is a doctoral student at Tulane University Graduate School of Social Work in New Orleans, Louisiana. Previously, she worked with the Family Advocacy, Care, and Educational Services (FACES) of Children's Hospital for ten years. This program delivered comprehensive social services and health education for HIV-positive women, children, youth, and their families in New Orleans. Contact information: <dgruber123@aol.com> or Tulane University, New Orleans.

Larry D. Icard, PhD, is the dean of the School of Social Administration at Temple University, Philadelphia, Pennsylvania. Dr. Icard can be reached at <Larry.Icard@Temple.edu>.

Lena Lundgren, PhD, is an associate professor of social policy at Boston University School of Social Work. She is also director of the Center on Work and Family. She is currently directing a three-year study on the service and drug treatment needs of IDUs. Dr. Lundgren also recently completed a three-year study to evaluate a multiyear community-level HIV prevention effort targeting 1,300 IDUs.

Kurt C. Organista, PhD, is an associate professor of social welfare at the University of California, Berkeley, and director of the Center for Latino Policy Research. He received his doctorate in clinical psychology from Arizona State University. He conducts Latino health and mental health research with an emphasis on HIV prevention in Mexican migrant laborers, and the treatment of depression in Latinos. He teaches courses on psychopathology (assessment and diagnosis), stress and coping, social work practice with Latinos, and human diversity. He currently serves on the editorial boards of the *Journal of Ethnic and Cultural Diversity in Social Work, Hispanic Journal of the Behavioral Sciences,* and the *American Journal of Community Psychology.*

San Patten <san.acch@shaw.ca> completed a MSc in community health sciences at the University of Calgary, specializing in the social context of HIV risk reduction behaviors among injection drug users. Upon completing her degree, San served as project leader at the AIDS Calgary Awareness Association where she was responsible for program planning, evaluation, and funding applications. Currently, San is working for the Alberta Community Council on HIV as a research technical assistant, building capacity among AIDS service organizations to conduct community-based research. San's interests include international health, human rights, harm reduction, program evaluation, and health research.

Peggy Pittman-Munke is on faculty at Murray State University in Murray, Kentucky. Her interests include the effects of welfare reform on persons of color and immigrants, social work history, domestic violence issues and undocumented immigrants, health issues and people of color, and distance learning. Her e-mail address is <pmunke@aol.com>.

Timothy Purington, MEd, is the director of harm reduction services at Tapestry Health Systems, Inc. At Tapestry Health he directs HIV/ HCV prevention programs for injection drug users, Hepatitis C services for recently infected individuals, HIV counseling and testing, syringe exchange, and oversees data gathering for a research collaboration with Boston University. He has served as a statewide consultant for the Massachusetts Department of Public Health concerning community planning for developing needle exchange programs. In 2000 he received the Ruth Batson Advocate of the Year Award from the Massachusetts Council of Human Service Providers.

Sybil G. Schroeder is an ABD student in the PhD program at Tulane University School of Social Work and is project director of the 2001-2002 Ryan White Title I Care Coordination Training for HIV/AIDS case managers and intake personnel in the New Orleans EMA through Southern University at New Orleans School of Social Work. She has practice experience in HIV/AIDS prevention services and resides in New Orleans, Louisiana. Ms. Schroeder can be reached at <sybilnola@ mindspring.com>.

Nushina Siddiqui is with the Center for Intervention and Practice Research at the School of Social Work, the University of Pennsylvania at Philadelphia.

Vincent J. Venturini, LCSW, is an assistant professor and field coordinator, Department of Criminal Justice and Social Work, Mississippi Valley State University, Itta Bena, Mississippi. He is currently a doctoral student at the University of Alabama School of Social Work and has many years of social work practice experience in rural areas.

Foreword

I consider writing the foreword to *Practice Issues in HIV/AIDS Services: Empowerment-Based Models and Program Applications* a distinct honor. Organized into eight chapters, the book leads the reader from a conceptual framework utilizing the generalist practice model to specific case studies focused mainly on the southern part of the United States. The first chapter by Mancoske and Smith, which is a foundation to the content of the following chapters, focuses specifically on approaches related to the ongoing HIV/AIDS crises in the United States and provides insights for practice related to challenges of the disease, modes of infection, special populations, psychosocial impact, treatment, and empowerment strategies. Likewise, this chapter incorporates the problem-solving approach to practice and provides the framework for culturally competent practice using case scenarios emphasizing empowerment from the initial data-gathering stage to termination. The importance of ethical practice is emphasized within the context of human rights and quality of life.

The second chapter by Gruber on case management provides an overview of case management approaches and emphasizes the importance of interdisciplinary teamwork to effectively and efficiently coordinate quality services for various complex needs. Best practices necessitate a continued partnership between practitioners and researchers. Gruber includes a thorough discussion of practice models of case management for persons living with HIV/AIDS, and covers emerging trends in the field, and service and research implications.

Although studies of the AIDS pandemic confirm the fact that sexual contact is the most common mode of transmission of HIV, it has been found that injection drug use is the second most common mode. Patton tackles this critical issue of injection drug use and transmission of HIV in Chapter 3 through an analysis of the transtheoretical model of behavior change for use with HIV/AIDS populations. According to Patten, the merit of this model is that it integrates several psychotherapeutic models into a comprehensive framework for explaining the underlying structure of behavior change and is a useful approach in working with "clients who are not ready to make active changes in their behaviors." It provides a perspective of health promotion that focuses on appropriate intervention that meets the needs of the individual during various stages of the change process.

Chapter 4 by Fitzgerald, Purington, Davis, Ferguson, and Lundgren explores the impact of injection drug use in substance abuse treatment and the spread of HIV infection. It is the one study in the book that focuses on areas beyond the southern part of the United States, incorporating data from Massachusetts where injection drug use is the leader in HIV transmission. The authors take a public health perspective in approaching drug abuse problems by promoting the philosophy of "harm reduction" referring to a "nonjudgmental approach to working with injection drug users." Furthermore, the findings, according to the authors, state that a substantial portion of injection drug users in the study care about their health, and were actively involved in reducing the harm related to their drug use through participation in needle exchange and substance abuse treatment programs. Practice implications suggest that social workers should understand that relapses and additional treatment episodes are often acceptable and necessary treatment paths for clients in their efforts to stop chronic drug addiction. Finally, the authors postulate that harm reduction permits social work practitioners to work with drug users while affirming that the users are the primary agents of reducing harm from their drug use, thereby empowering users and embracing the social work value of "meeting the client where he or she is."

In Chapter 5 Kurt Organista discusses the HIV/AIDS epidemic and the inefficient preventive measures regarding the poverty-stricken, isolated, and uninsured among Mexican migrant farmworkers in the United States. Later in the chapter, he recommends strategies to improve prevention rates and treatment modalities with special emphasis on education related to HIV/AIDS, condom distribution, culturally specific knowledge, and empowering strategies. Policy implications related to change in federal laws for migrant farmworkers include improving "farmworker wages, employee benefits, and health- and safety-related working conditions."

Icard and Siddiqui discuss family-based interventions with African-American underserved populations. The authors focus on the important issue of reaching these populations through family-focused HIV interventions with special emphasis on the family change agent who is the target of intervention, and the focal family member whose behavior is influenced by the family change agent. The authors provide notable examples of family-focused approaches to interventions with African Americans with the guiding premise that behavioral change remains the only means for primary prevention of HIV. The concept of hidden populations encompasses hard-to-reach populations of African Americans that are significantly diverse in composition and values and involve biological, legal, social, and emotional relationships and commitments. Moreover, the authors note the need to assess the application of theoretical models for use as guides in work to reduce the prevalence of HIV/AIDS among these groups. Finally, they suggest both ongoing evaluation of practice and research in the prevention of HIV/AIDS.

In Chapter 7 Pittman-Munke and Venturini present an overview of the HIV/AIDS conditions among African Americans in the Mississippi and Louisiana Delta. Due in part to poverty, high unemployment, low education, and embedded religious and social conditions that stigmatize the HIV/AIDS population, the rate of HIV infection in this region is one of the highest in the United States. The authors discuss the significance of cultural tradition and the prime stature of the organized church in the region. Continuing the use of the generalist model as the backdrop for community practice, the authors emphasize a strengths-based approach to practice combining the knowledge, values, and role of the church and HIV/AIDS communities in the Delta. This strategy incorporates a best practices model for both treatment-oriented services and for primary prevention, thus providing a holistic approach for reaching the targeted communities.

In Chapter 8 Schroeder examines the status of the HIV/ AIDS epidemic among African-American women in Louisiana. After providing statistics on HIV/AIDS in African-American communities in Louisiana, she argues that they should not be viewed as homogenous and that research and practice strategies should take into account the prevailing social, cultural, and economic conditions of the specific community.

A critical review of this book indicates that the topics covered are extremely important today and in the foreseeable future for social work practice and for use by other human services and health professionals. Its emphasis on the unique aspects of practice that speak to special populations, considering culture, gender, and geographic issues within the context of generalist practice and the problem-solving method also makes it an excellent reference for practitioners, educators, and students. The book skillfully interweaves theory and practice, recommending new approaches or strengthening existing ones. Each chapter is supported by extensive use of pertinent sources, solid methodologies, and sound conclusions.

Gwendolyn Spencer Prater
Dean and Professor of Social Work
Jackson State University
School of Social Work

Chapter 1

A Generalist Practice Model in HIV/AIDS Services: An Empowerment Perspective

Ronald J. Mancoske
James Donald Smith

THE ONGOING CHALLENGES OF HIV/AIDS

Although AIDS-related mortalities are declining in the United States, new and increasing HIV infections continue to create life-threatening challenges. HIV may be described as a series of epidemics impacting diverse populations in unique ways, creating special populations with unique threats and burdens. These may be described as "rebound epidemics." Some changes have helped limit increasing infections in some populations, whereas other areas are reporting rebounding infection rates. Although the incidence of HIV infections has stabilized, the increasing survival pattern means people infected tend to be surviving longer, which challenges the care delivery systems as more people live with chronic HIV infections (Lee, Karon, and Selik, 2001). The impacts of new infections have caused many persons living with HIV/AIDS (PWAs) to require assistance in coping with the psychosocial sequalae to HIV/AIDS. These challenges change as new medical treatments change the overall course of HIV disease and the biopsychosocial impacts of this persisting life-threatening disease. The generalist model focus of this book examines common problems and experiences not only by identification of problems and possible solutions, but also by building on the strengths which are drawn upon to confront the challenges of HIV/AIDS.

The Pathways of HIV

Although new HIV/AIDS treatments continue to advance, the cost remains high. The National Institutes for Health spent approximately $1.7 billion for research in 1997 (Nathanson, 1998). Spending rises every year. Even with triple-drug therapy costing more than $6,000 per person annually, these costs still remain less than treatment of other illnesses. Globally, more than 40 million people have HIV/AIDS, and HIV infection rates are rising beyond belief, mostly in the poorest regions of the world (United Nations Economic and Social Council, 2002). The United Nations group report states that the epidemic has been grossly underestimated, and that we are in just the beginning of the pandemic. In the early twenty-first century, some countries are reporting more than one-third of their adult populations infected. The international implications of this are far more devastating than early projects implied (Mancoske, 1997a). This is a plague that has been predicted (Garrett, 1994) and will be far worse than anything history has visited upon us.

The Presidential Advisory Council on HIV/AIDS (2000) notes that in the United States over 400,000 individuals have died from AIDS and another 700,000 to 900,000 persons are living with HIV infection. Approximately 40,000 new cases of HIV infection are reported annually—a figure stabilizing after explosive growth in the prior decade ("The Public Health Challenges of the HIV Epidemic," 2000). The highest rates of infections remain in less developed nations where the results of these advances in treatment remain beyond the reach of all but a few—and thus the progression to death remains quick and sure for many (Mancoske, 1997a). Although some hope remains with vaccines that are being tested in humans, the time lines for getting the vaccines to people in general may take years, and thus the hope remains with prevention. Due to new strains of the virus developing and resistence to the new treatments remaining a major concern, the challenges remain vast. In the meantime, many will continue to be impacted by HIV/AIDS. The survival time after an AIDS diagnosis is increasing. A report indicates that in 1984 those diagnosed on average lived less than a year from the time of diagnosis. Beginning in the mid-1990s, the survival rate on average was at least three years (Lee, Karon, and Selik, 2001). Many persons in the United States are living longer, and with quality and effective care and supports, they have dramatically improved their quality of life.

HIV and Special Populations

The HIV epidemic increasingly affects women, minorities, persons infected through heterosexual contact, and the poor (Karon et al., 2001). The HIV epidemic has always had disparate impacts on various populations. It was initially misnomered as GRID (Gay-Related Immune Deficiency) in the early 1980s because of the initial impact first found among urban gay male populations (Shilts, 1987). The numbers of gay and bisexual men infected with HIV remain stable—similar levels were reported from 1989 through 1998 (HIV/AIDS Bureau, 2000). However, analysis of epedimiological data from 1994 to 2000 suggests a resurgence of HIV incidence among men who have sex with men. Men who have sex with other men remain the leading HIV exposure category of new cases in the United States, although only slightly so in 2001 (CDC, 2001).

In 2002, the number of AIDS cases in the world (United Nations Economic and Social Council, 2002) was estimated to be more than 40 million people, with 43 percent of infections among women (Fauci, 2000). Fauci estimated that 16,000 new infections would occur each day. More than 23 percent of new cases reported in 1998 in the United States were among women (HIV/AIDS Bureau, 2000). By mid-2001, the Centers for Disease Control and Prevention (2001) estimated 139,217 female AIDS cases diagnosed in the United States. By 2000, nearly 11,000 HIV diagnoses of children were reported to the CDC (National Abandoned Infants Resource Center, 2002). Between 6,000 and 7,000 HIV-positive women in the United States give birth each year with infections of infants at about 30 percent unless the mother is in treatment, where infections then are at about 8 percent (CDC, 2000). Most of these pediatric cases are among African-American women (62 percent) and 90 percent of these infected children rely on Medicaid for health care services. Approximately 10 percent of the United States population of persons living with HIV are over fifty years of age, and of these, older women appear to have higher incidences of infections (United Nations Global AIDS Program, 2002).

The overall epidemic in the United States might best be viewed as a number of distinct subepidemics existing among women, minorities, injection drug users and their partners, gays, heterosexuals, and adolescents (Nathanson, 1998). The most effective prevention and intervention strategies require careful planning for each special population. Early strategies to confront the epidemic focused on public education and assumed that everyone was at risk. However, it remains true that some are considerably more at risk for various social, economic, cultural, and other reasons and thus special populations require special services. It has been controversial to focus on special populations of the epidemic in part because of the stigma associated with AIDS (Sontag, 1988). The founder and principal architect of early world AIDS programs, Jonathan Mann, convincingly taught that all AIDS work must focus on stigma reduction and human rights—an empowerment emphasis (1997). Advocacy is an essential component of empowerment-based generalist practice. Catania and colleagues (2001) examined epidemiological data on HIV infections in the United States urban areas and concluded that although HIV prevalence appears to be declining from the mid-1980s overall, in segments of the population (men who have sex with men, African Americans, injection drug users, and the less educated), infection levels are catastrophically high and comparable to sub-Saharan Africa levels. A related report shows a reversal of trends with increases in current gonorrhea cases among men who have sex with men (Fox et al., 2001) which can be considered a marker of increasing HIV infections.

By the end of 1998, there were between 650,000 and 900,000 persons in the United States infected with HIV (HIV/AIDS Bureau, 2000). In 1998, more than 66 percent of new cases were among racial and ethnic minorities. Mortality has declined less among minorities and women than among white males. The report notes that infections are eight times greater among African Americans than among whites, and that men of color represent 45 percent of new infections among gay and bisexual men (HIV/AIDS Bureau, 2000). A *Washington Blade* article ("CDC: Gay, Bisexual Men Driving Epidemic," 1999), citing the CDC data, notes that the new infections among black gay and bisexual men are largely driving the AIDS epidemic in some African-American communities. The article notes that the surgeon general reported that 70 percent of the new cases of HIV infections identified from July 1999 to June 2000 were among African Americans and Hispanics. The report further notes epidemiological data showing that African-American females comprise three out of five new female infections, with most of these women having young children. An article in *The New York Times* ("Undeterred by a monster," 2001) reported on a study of young men who have sex with other men in New York City. The study found 33 percent of the African-American men sampled to be HIV positive, 16 percent of the men overall, and 2 percent of the white men. The report attributed the high infection rates among African-American young men to "secrecy, stigma, and youthful folly."

Half of new infections over the past several years have been among those ages thirteen to twenty-four (White House Report, 2000). This report notes that most youth who are already infected do not know they are infected and few receive medical care. One-fourth of all new infections in 1998 were reported to be among youths (under twenty-one years of age), especially those that are homeless, victims of abuse, and sexual minorities. The rate of new infections among African Americans and Hispanic Americans is increasing four times faster for African Americans and two times faster for Hispanic Americans than among the overall population increases (Dean, Fleming, and Ward, 1993). Risk for HIV infection of women is not evenly distributed—some are more at risk than others. Racial and ethnic minority women are at higher risk for becoming infected by their male partners. Incarcerated women upon release may face enhanced risks of unprotected sex and injection drug use because of social, emotional, and economic circumstances. The power dynamics in interpersonal relationships and processes of negotiating for safer sex combine with other higher female risks for infection. Pregnancies for at-risk women combined with access barriers to care add to at-risk vulnerabilities.

Women are increasingly being infected with HIV. AIDS cases among females have increased from 6.7 percent in 1986 to 18 percent in 1999 (McKeown, 2001). McKeown states that women now account for nearly one-quarter of all new AIDS cases diagnosed and 32 percent of new reported infections. Women living in Southern states, particularly African-American women, are becoming infected at alarming rates, especially in some rural Southern areas. Many of these women are infected through no readily identifiable risk other than heterosexual contact. Internationally, female infections increased to 47 percent of new infections (Kaiser Family Foundation, 2002). In the United States, women comprise 23 percent of all AIDS cases and women of color account for 77 percent of all women diagnosed (National Abandoned Infants Resource Center, 2002).

AIDS cases reflect a time period ranging from initial infection until an AIDS diagnosis is made. This may camouflage increasing rates of HIV infections among women, especially impoverished African-American women. In a 1998 report on studies of federal Job Corps applicants over the prior five years, Bynum (1998) reported that the rate of infection among applicant women ages sixteen to twenty-one was 50 percent higher than that of men in the same group. The highest rates were among African-American females, with five out of every 1,000 applicants infected with HIV. This in part might be attributed to the fact that young women tend to have sexual relations with men who are a bit older than themselves, thus increasing infection risk. These young women are being infected at nearly twice the rate of young men.

Cornelius Baker of the Whitman-Walker Clinic in Washington, DC, believes that many African-American women are infected by men who "secretly" have sex with other men (Sternberg, 2001). Many African-American men may engage in sex with men, but do not consider themselves gay, and thus they do not believe they are susceptible to HIV because they believe gay identity is synonymous with "white." Baker believes this explains why two-thirds of female AIDS cases are among African-American women. Higher incidence of sexually transmitted diseases increases the risk for HIV infection, which may also account for the high rate of infection (Sternberg, 2001). Women of color also tend not to be receiving antiretroviral therapy because of drug use, risky sexual behavior, depression, and unmet social needs that interfere with medical access.

In the early 1990s, the incidence of HIV infections was being reported as three times higher among Hispanics than among whites (Diaz et al., 1993). The incidence of AIDS cases in mid-2000 totaled 20 percent of the reported cases (CDC, 2001). The incidence rates vary widely among exposure categories based on countries of origin for Hispanics. Injection drug use constitutes a larger portion of new cases than found in the general population, except for lower incidence among Hispanic women. These data indicate unique programming needs targeting prevention, early intervention, and ongoing service needs.

Of the 40 million people in the world living with HIV, it is estimated that 38 percent are youths under twenty-five years of age (Kaiser Family Foundation, 2002). Kaiser reports that 58 percent of new infections are among youths. Youth AIDS deaths are reversing life expectancy in many countries. In the United States, many of the infected youths tend to be difficult to reach because they are often not in school nor among the formally employed. Adolescents comprise the fastest growing group of new HIV infections (National Abandoned Infants Resource Center, 2002). Although youths nationally comprise less than 1 percent of the diagnosed cases of AIDS (Louisiana Office of Public Health, 1998), more infections occur among youths. According to reports from the Centers for Disease Control and Prevention, 48 percent of youths were sexually active with 16 percent having more than four partners, and 33 percent engaged in binge drinking within the prior month ("Teenagers at Risk," 1998). Youths worldwide tend to be increasingly at risk because they do not perceive themselves at risk, have high rates of other sexually transmitted diseases, and live in the broader context of poverty (Kaiser Family Foundation, 2002). This occurs in a climate in which sex education for youth is not provided universally nor systematically. In 1997, 50 percent of the estimated 40,000 new HIV infections were among persons under age twenty-five (Sternberg, 1998). The majority (58 percent) of these youths were African Americans (Texeira, 1998).

HIV infection rates are particularly high in prisons where most inmates represent ethnic minorities. The HIV rate in prisons is five times greater than among the general population (Office of Minority Health, 2001). This poses multiple challenges given the diverse agendas of corrections compared with public health.

A wide variation of infection rates exists depending upon geographic locations. First identified in urban areas, the epidemic is increasing in rural areas. Although the number of new cases are leveling off in urban areas, they are increasing in rural areas, particularly in the rural South (Mankoske, 1997b). The vulnerabilities of rural persons include risks such as social and geographic isolation, maldistribution of medical and care resources, higher rates of poverty than in urban areas in general, and other sociocultural features (Smith and Mancoske, 1997). Infections are contracted by a diversity of routes of transmission, including men who have sex with men, injection drug use, and heterosexual transmission. Given uniqueness and problems with health and social service delivery in rural areas, many questions emerge over in-migration and out-migration for care access. Barriers to care and isolation characterize the experiences of rural PWAs.

Access to care for special populations must be examined because less than optimal care contributes to disparities in outcomes and to a disproportionate distribution of suffering. In a national sample, Shapiro et al. (1999) reported that African Americans, Latinos, women, the uninsured, and those receiving Medicaid tended to have less desirable patterns of care access. These patterns need to be reversed if this pandemic is to be controlled and costs for treatment contained. In order to prevent HIV infections, secure early interventions in care planning, and provide services to those with HIV/AIDS, it becomes imperative to consider the uniqueness of the experiences of special populations impacted by HIV. Continued discussion of special populations is necessary.

Psychosocial Aspects of HIV/AIDS

Life-threatening illness impacts the well-being of those affected by AIDS. Physical health, psychological health, and social well-being interactionally impact one another, and problems in one area have identifiable effects on other areas. Psychosocial risk impacts illness progression and the extent of one's physical health, although the exact mechanisms are often unclear (Rayner-Brosnan, 1995). From a systems perspective, it is necessary to examine interactions at all systems levels (individual, family, groups, organizations, and communities) as these impact health and well-being.

Psychosocial risks common to various persons who live with HIV/AIDS are affected by social supports, psychosocial adjustments, psychological distress, substance use, the social impact of disease on family and social status, and risk-taking behaviors. The severity level of the disease impacts the level of psychosocial distress, causing varying needs at different points in the life of the disease (Chuang et al., 1989). Persons living with HIV/AIDS face common challenges, including emotional problems, suicidal feelings, uncertainty, relationship problems, and interpersonal issues related to infections. Some common needs center around managing stress, self-esteem, social isolation, decision making, disclosure, and family relations (Dilley, Pies, and Helquist, 1993). Persons who better manage biopsychosocial aspects of HIV/AIDS have improved health outcomes.

The psychosocial impact of HIV on family systems did not receive considerable attention in the first decade of the epidemic, in part because HIV was considered a gay-related phenomenon, which was compounded by the general low level of cultural competence among service providers working with gay men and lesbian women and their families (Holmes and Hodge, 1995). HIV causes problems in family dynamics and family structures, problems with loss and grief, and family problems related to other social systems (Bor and Miller, 1988). These issues are essential components of family assessments. Although these dynamics appear to be influenced by HIV in affected families, they differ according to the various dynamic levels found in families (Bonuck, 1993). The family's developmental level influences coping strategies for the stress of illness. Younger children tend to grapple more with issues of separation whereas teens tend to deal more with symptoms related to anger control (Mellins and Ehrhardt, 1994). Social and interactional problems may occur with other institutions such as medical care delivery systems, child care, schools, extended families, and social service agencies.

Families of gay men may have problems with disclosure issues, role differentiation, or emotional distance (McMillan, 1988). Women infected with HIV who have children cope with problems such as planning for the long-term care of the children, barriers to access, and connections with care. Many of these women are single parents or in unstable relationships with men, and face problems with histories of substance abuse, domestic violence, and economic deprivation, which in turn contribute to feelings of isolation, fear, and estrangement from parenting challenges. Welfare policies have made it clear that women cannot depend upon financial assistance for long-term structural poverty conditions. Social work practice models provide inroads into the problem-solving process in working with families with HIV/AIDS, although the needs of these families often outpace the capacities of helpers to meet them (Talyor-Brown and Garcia, 1995).

The HIV/AIDS stigma threatens group status and identity. It promotes isolation and estrangement from families and other groups. It poses barriers to group participation—from assuming a sick role to assuming a damaged identity. Group dynamics offer critical issues to examine in the helping process (Mancoske and Lindhorst, 1994). Support groups have been particularly effective in helping women cope with cancer and to improve the quality of life of those suffering from life-threatening illnesses. Such groups provide similar help in HIV/AIDS care.

Living with HIV/AIDS generally brings persons into contact with formal organizations, which for some might be the first time they need extensive major medical care or social services. Many social service organizations have been developed to provide care and services. These are often funded by federal government allocations to Medicare, Medicaid, or via Ryan White CARE Act funds. These organizations often develop specializations in AIDS care. Service providers in HIV/AIDS services organizations (ASOs) face common challenges in dealing with the stigma of HIV work. The challenges of this complex interdisciplinary work include the devaluation in working with poor persons and cultural minorities, the political climate that marginalizes work with sexual minorities, and dependence upon medical research and specialized practice (Wilson, 1995).

Changing community opinions have influenced the new rash of legislation in such areas as partner notification, criminal sanctions for putting others at risk, and disclosing data on infections. These changes are influenced by public health concerns, conservative social climates, and a backlash to earlier approaches. Fears persist that current policies will keep people away from services. Service providers at the community level often are concerned with establishing strong coalitions, empowering affected groups in self-care, developing working groups that confront barriers to care, linking to diverse groups, and promoting interdisciplinary working groups.

Access to quality care is a formidable issue for many persons living with HIV/AIDS. Only one-half to one-third of HIV-positive persons receive care, and access barriers influence this. The HIV/AIDS Bureau (2000) reported that 20 percent of those in care had no public or private insurance, 29 percent were enrolled in Medicaid, 32 percent had private insurance, 72 percent had incomes less than $25,000 and 46 percent had incomes less than $10,000 annually, and 63 percent were unemployed. The report indicated that women are not only poorer than men, but in one area, 30 percent of the women had average incomes of less than $5,000 annually. As infection rates continue to increase among poor women and minorities, these access barriers increase.

Social work practitioners need to be aware of the unique vulnerabilities of special populations to HIV/AIDS to effectively target specific interventions for them. Although it was known in the early 1980s that HIV would not be containable among urban gay male populations, it was not until the second decade of the epidemic that this became a clear focal point of intervention plans. Social workers comprise the single largest provider of mental health services to persons with HIV and thus are at the front lines of service delivery (Lynch, Lloyd, and Fimbres, 1993). It is imperative to recognize the changing face of AIDS and what to do about the unique needs and stigma management among special populations.

In summary, vulnerabilities of special populations require an advocacy stance for the provision of services to those most at risk for HIV. Strategies that empower those at risk offer the most hope in the complex dynamics of controlling the HIV epidemic and increasing access to quality health care. Improved access requires effective service outreach to vulnerable populations. Case management models should be chosen to improve access at all system levels. A variety of case management models exist. Generalist practice models with an empowerment perspective call for core functions such as data gathering, assessment, planning interventions, information and referral, case advocacy, providing a treatment plan, evaluating service outcomes, and appropriate terminations. In some cases, a limited brokerage case management model is adequate, but this is not a comprehensive case management approach which is generally indicated in effective HIV services.

The Role of Advancing Medical Treatments in HIV Care

The news reports from the International AIDS Conference in 1997 bristled with excitement as the new evidence of success of the drug cocktails began to come to eager and often demoralized conferees and communities watching for treatment progress. New hope arose for those struggling with limited treatments for the heretofore "uniformly fatal disease" when they heard the news indicating that mortality rates for AIDS were declining. An article in *The Washington Post* ("No AIDS Obits," 1998) reported that the gay weekly *Bay Area*

Reporter reported no AIDS deaths that week, marking the first time in seventeen years that the paper had not had AIDS-related deaths to report. AIDS-related obituaries began declining in 1996. San Francisco reported thirty-five AIDS deaths in July 1998, down from 150 deaths in July 1992. Medical claims for insurance coverage of AIDS treatments dropped to less than $1 billion in 1997, the first time in nine years that the total claims were less than $1 billion (Levin, 1998a).

Press reports were more cautious after the 1998 International AIDS Conference. One Associated Press medical editor reported that 30 to 60 percent of all people taking the new drug combinations were "treatment failures." The drugs did not reduce viral levels, or if they did, people experienced a rebound of the virus, usually in a different form (Haney, 1998). For many, the new treatments offered the sought-after "magic bullet," but with the uncertainty of how long they would last, whether they would create side effects that might also be lethal, or whether a new drug-resistant strain of the virus might rapidly develop. The exuberance of declining death rates was complicated by medical decisions about when best to start treatments, which treatment types to prescribe, and how long to continue treatment regimens with uncertain outcomes. Thus, persons living with HIV may have complex interactions with medical care providers necessitating information and choices that are clearly life-and-death defining. The perception that AIDS can be treated with medications may also cause a reduction in prevention efforts in some communities, contributing to a rebound in new infections.

Wide disparity exists in access to HIV treatments. James (2000) reported on a study examining four states, noting that half to two-thirds of persons relying on public care failed to receive proper treatment. Many of the patients were unable to obtain needed medications through Medicaid or state drug assistance programs. Fifty-four percent of persons with HIV who are receiving treatment are enrolled in managed care systems (Link, 1999). Link argues that no governmental program is more important to persons with HIV than Medicaid, which is moving toward greater levels of managed care with its inherently contradictory policies that impact HIV-care access. Optimal treatment depends largely on locale and access to coverage. Living in rural areas and in the South appears to be a significant risk factor for being untreated and for having inadequate access to medications or psychosocial services (James, 2000). In urban impoverished areas where access is particularly difficult, various targeted access approaches have been attempted: reaching the homeless and marginally housed, as well as those with addictions, mental illness, and individuals ensnared in persistent poverty. These urban groups are less likely to be treated with current effective medications and treatment advances (Bamberger et al., 2000). Bamberger and colleagues recommend aggressive outreach using storefront centers. Evidence of successful treatments has been found with this approach. E-mail has been used with a few of the participants for follow-up when possible and cost-effective benefits of early intervention and appropriate medical treatments have been reported.

One of the major issues of treatment success is adherence to complex medication regimens. In 1997, the new guidelines for HIV therapy were issued and in a study of people in treatment, S. Levin (1998) reported that 70 percent were receiving the recommended triple-drug therapy. Successes in treatments deserve optimism, although they do add various other concerns to care planning. For example, it becomes necessary for persons to make informed decisions about when to begin medications, which ones, and for how long. This requires informed participation in complex and uncertain medical procedures. It requires a basic sense of trust between providers and consumers. Concerns persist that HMOs might not provide optimal care but are cost-effective—both having potentially differing consequences. Persons who at one time needed to obtain permanent disability benefits quickly now have to reassess when and how to best make these preparations. This may include help with planning for psychosocial aspects of long-term care and social supports.

In a study of treatment failures at Veterans Affairs Medical Centers, a strong parallel was established between successful outcomes and treatment adherence (Paterson, Swindells, and Mohr, 2000). Those persons receiving optimal treatments and who complied with medical interventions had consistently positive health outcomes. Ways to improve adherence were studied, including targeting those with mental illness for specialized interventions that enhance adherence (Paterson, Swindells, and Mohr, 2000). Programs developed to encourage adherence often focus on the psychosocial sequalae of HIV infection; when these problems are resolved, adherence improves (Shelton, 2000). Peer group supports are recommended to deal with such problems as complications of drug regimens, viral rebounds, changing therapies, drug holidays (periods without the drugs), side effects of medications, drug resistence, addictions, and despair. Peer support groups provide an effective mechanism for enhancing adherence. The *Houston Chronicle* reported on studies at a local HIV clinic showing that 80 percent of patients took the medications improperly (Hooper, 2000). The researchers characterized adherence to be "dismal." In a national study, Andersen and colleagues (2000) found that African Americans, injection drug users, women, and people with limited education were least likely to receive the benefits of optimal treatments. Optimal interventions are becoming more effective, and more vulnerable groups are less likely to receive optimal treatments, and these treatments are more likely to be delayed. Improving access not only enhances health outcomes, but evidence shows that it is cost effective as well. Increasing spending on optimal treatments saves overall medical intervention costs (Tolson, 2000).

Adherence and optimal treatments lead to greatly improved health outcomes in HIV. In a booklet prepared to promote adherence, Bartlett (2000) cites research from various sources to summarize known ways to promote adherence in HIV treatments. He cites first a number of processes to enhance adherence: assess readiness for treatment, assess barriers, intervene with affective disorders or substance use disorders, develop family supports where appropriate, keep prescription practices as simple as possible, and mix interventions to promote adherence (education, peer supports, follow-ups, etc.). Bartlett (2000) also offers evidence of what works best to promote adherence, such as pill boxes, written instructions, and simpler medication regimens. Adherence may be misunderstood within complicated treatment decision areas, such as when structured therapeutic interruptions are recommended.

Early intervention means providing treatments immediately following exposure to the virus. Some advocate for a "hit hard, hit early" strategy, although this strategy also poses risks. The risks include developing drug-resistant strains and viral mutations that may not respond to treatments in the long run. Many persons are kept alive for years, but it is unknown at which point medications may cease effectiveness and no other medications may work in their stead. Thus, some discussions of drug holidays and other approaches further complicate medication regimens. More medications continue to enter the "pipeline" and make it possible to continue to try new treatments.

This requires sophisticated treatment planning and care coverage for new and changing treatments. Some are insured and are protected, others are not, and those dependent upon public funding are at the mercy of various social, economic, and policy constraints. Early interventions in pediatric cases minimize risk of perinatal transmission. Cesarean section deliveries prevent pediatric infections and combinational therapies for pregnant women offer evidence of positive outcomes (Cadman, 1998). Yet up to one-third of all HIV-positive individuals remain unaware of their serostatus, and receive no treatment at all (HIV/AIDS Bureau, 2000). The HIV/AIDS Bureau (2000) report also noted that as many as 200,000 Americans know they are HIV positive but received substandard care and as recently as 1998 less than half of those with HIV had been treated with the new antiretroviral medications. Some may choose not to be tested because of the stigma associated with being diagnosed and identified as having HIV/AIDS. The CDC *Mortality and Morbidity Weekly Report* described "a resurgent HIV epidemic among men who have sex with men" ("HIV Incidence Among Young Men," 2001, p. 44).

Some critical issues in care delivery have important influences on access to care as well as care outcomes. A *New York Times* article reported that a growing body of research indicated that, in general, more health care may not necessarily be better (Kolata, 2002). However, research demonstrates that better access to care improves survival time after an AIDS diagnosis (Montgomery et al., 2002). Having a regular source of AIDS care enhances survivability. Based on evidence from Ryan White CARE Act service recipients, the HIV/AIDS Bureau (2000) suggests seven critical aspects to current care:

1. *provider training and experience:* many providers lack essential training and experience;
2. *care in underserved areas:* most individuals needing care are coming now from these areas;
3. *comprehensive care:* most individuals now have multiple diagnoses and live in poverty;
4. *HIV-positive individuals are not in care:* poverty, stigma, multiple problems, and lack of information all contribute to the fact that over a third do not even know their HIV status;
5. *quantifiable outcome data:* better systems of tracking care and outcomes are needed;

6. *treatment and adherence:* adherence to care needs to be improved; and
7. *health insurance and financing:* eligibility and access barriers are great.

Questions of who gets into early treatment, and who follows optimal treatment strategies, often means that there are less concerns with the development of drug resistence. The new treatments are characterized by the development of drug resistence (Gilden, Falkenberg, and Torres, 1997). One study reported that at least half of the patients in one clinic experienced drug resistence (Stephenson, 2002). Recognition of and interventions for substance use problems are important to care, but low-level screening and interventions are a general problem in health care delivery (Friedmann, McCullough, and Saitz, 2001). At optimal compliance are concerns about developing resistance to the medications and the emergence of new strains of the virus. The medical treatments are complex and challenging and individuals with a host of other problems, including alcohol and drug problems, dementia, depression, or relationship crises may find adherence more difficult to achieve.

Some persons develop complications associated with new therapies. These may not be readily treatable and may require that treatment be suspended in some cases. For example, lipodystrophy syndrome (central fat accumulation, depletion, or metabolic disturbance), can result from medication. These situations have immense bearing on psychosocial conditions such as self-esteem, self-image, problems with social or sexual relations, threats to locus of control, forced HIV disclosure, demoralization, or depression (Collins, Wagner, and Walmsley, 2000).

The complex role of vaccine development has yet to play its potential major role in the worldwide HIV pandemic (Cohen, 2001). New vaccines are being tested on volunteers and within a few years, reports should help clarify their role in prevention and treatment. Vaccine use may interact with various other social, economic, and behavioral dynamics. For example, vaccines may increase HIV seroprevalence if condom use declines or if vaccines are not cost effective in penetrating at-risk areas (Edwards, Shachter, and Owens, 1998). A great many medical concerns become entwined in a broad array of social and economic issues. Effective problem-solving interventions offer potential to promote optimal medical care, improved public health, and improved psychosocial functioning.

Guidelines for medical interventions change rapidly as science and knowledge dissemination evolves. Thus, new questions are continually raised and assumptions made about such basic issues as when to start treatments, what treatments to start, how to promote adherence to best practices, and which interventions promote the best results. Optimal outcomes require current best practices in medical interventions combined with best practices in psychosocial interventions. This becomes a major navigational challenge through care systems for persons with complex barriers to adequate medical and social supports. From an empowerment perspective, care providers must keep abreast of changing evidence-based practice guidelines, and this information must be shared with persons making the complex choices for self-care that promote health and well-being.

An Empowerment Perspective in Generalist Practice

Despite the widespread negative valuation placed on many of the special populations vulnerable to the impact of HIV, these persons do not interact uniformly in social environments. Some persons find personal, social, and other resources to counteract this negative valuation (Solomon, 1976). Those who can best mobilize personal and social resources to confront the challenges will do best at all systems levels. Empowerment practice uses generalist problem-solving models with a focus on issues of power and strengths in transactions, at micro, mezzo, and macro levels.

Persons living with HIV/AIDS (PWAs) may benefit from help in addressing a range of psychosocial challenges and barriers to optimal functioning. Conversely, PWAs are critical sources of energy in the struggle to develop programs and services for themselves. At times, individuals may require various services or the skills of professional care advocates to achieve improved functioning. Discrimination or intrapersonal feelings may impede individuals from taking steps to improve themselves and achieve their goals. This may require group-level interventions, especially when problems are interactional such as in dealing with service bureaucracies. At other times, the challenges involve addressing social policy areas impacting communities such as linkage development and networking. When persons feel involved in their own care and their own services, they take responsibility for themselves, their care, and the needs of others with similar concerns. Intercession in confronting these barriers to participation and self-care decision making may be indicated until individuals can and do become their own best advocates. When capacities are diminished because of physical or mental health reasons, professional intervention may become more important in developing social networks.

The generalist approach requires a scientific method applied to problem identification and problem solving. An empowerment approach does not limit itself to a problem focus but encourages a strengths perspective. Individual skills and resources are identified not only to help individuals resolve their own problems but also to develop strategies for empowering others with similar concerns. If the focus of care centers on individual problems, clinical treatment is indicated. If the focus involves individuals helping others with similar needs, the focus shifts to an empowerment perspective (Mancoske and Hunzeker, 1990). The empowerment perspective does not ignore individual difficulties—it promotes multiple system-level changes. Individuals are impacted but the focus expands to shared needs, shared resources, and service connections. Community empowerment is enhanced when there are no rivalries between service providers for special populations. Service integration is coordinated so that the unique and individual needs of all are competently addressed.

Hence, empowerment may involve individual, family, and/or group-level interventions that seek to promote social (policy, agency, and community level) changes. Just as individual service providers may feel overwhelmed by the suffering and the problems encountered in fighting the impact of disease and poverty, agency responses may also exhibit signs of hopelessness and helplessness. Brown (1996) describes how one agency achieves empowerment of staff and clients by emphasizing self-awareness, self-responsibility, commitment, inner guidance, and by manifesting desirable outcomes.

Services that empower vulnerable community groups emphasize advocacy, social action, education, outreach, and self-care. Prevention and education materials reflect the language and skills found in targeted communities. Collective community action is the focus. When working with special populations particularly vulnerable to social oppression and stigma, care should include an emphasis on problem solving from an empowerment perspective. Practitioners must develop competencies specific to the historical experiences of the risk groups they serve. Services should vigilantly track quality of life; service satisfaction; locus of control; the roles of family and kin; language and communication; spirituality; and roles and stereotypes in communities. Alternative explanations are required in the relationship-building process of generalist practice. Where particular vulnerabilities exist, and strategies are addressed to minimize them, change can be evaluated through working relationships.

GENERALIST PRACTICE MODEL

This section discusses the application of the generalist model to work with HIV/AIDS. It explicates some of the assumptions of this work.

Ecological Systems Theory

The use of a generalist practice model is based on the broad systems theory framework. The general systems theory addresses the expansive understanding of the person in situation. It reflects social work's traditional concerns with individual change as well as change in the social environment in which the individual acts and is acted upon. The ecological model translates this abstract systems language into a practice language more useful to applications (Germain and Gitterman, 1995). Practice requires workers to be familiar with multiple system levels and how they interact (Meyer and Mattaini, 1995). The system levels include: individuals, groups, couples, families, neighborhoods, formal and informal organizations, communities, and societies. Data gathering normally includes a review of the interactions between key problem areas and strengths at all system levels.

Generalist Practice Model Application

The generalist model is the application of the scientific problem-solving process at various system levels. This model focuses on working with changing systems at all levels, and is defined in different ways. This discussion of problem solving is based on relationship building, data gathering, assessing, intervening, evaluating, and terminating services (Mancoske and Hunzeker, 1990). Recent generalist texts provide variation on this same generalist model. Meyer and Mattaini (1995) describe the process as engagement, exploration, assessment, intervention, monitoring, maintenance, and termination. Hoffman and Sallee (1993) cite the process as identifying areas of concern and engagement, information gathering, assessing, planning and implementing change, evaluating, and developing transitions. Johnson (1988) provides a different discussion by noting interactions, assessment, planning, action, evaluation, and termination. McMahon (1995) discusses areas of engagement, data collection, assessment, intervention, evaluation, and termination. Using an empowerment approach in the generalist model, Miley, O'Melia, and Dubois (1998) define phases as follows: the dialogue phase (building relationships and assessing challenges), the discovery phase (assessing resources and planning change), and the developing phase (implementing, evaluating, and stabilizing change). Case management models built upon the generalist approach often use the same definitions as Rothman and Sager (1998): intake, assessment, goal setting, resource identification and intervention planning, therapy, linking, monitoring, evaluation, and advocacy.

Social work roles and functions in HIV/AIDS services can use a case management model, which is basically the generalist model applied to multiple system levels. Case management is the tool that can help PWAs access effective and cost-controlled services addressing a wide range of needs and programming. It is based on the assumption of a model that integrates physical, psychological, and social problems and strengths. Services are expected to be delivered based on related standards (Sowell and Meadows, 1994).

Case management is generalist practice that is less focused on treatment approaches and more focused on interdisciplinary, community-based, and multidimensional models of care. The models often are based on the cooperation of multidisciplinary interests on behalf of the PWA. Thus, with more of a community approach than a clinical approach, community-based interventions are less likely to be ignored (Goodman et al., 1996). Goodman and colleagues discuss community interventions and evaluation of services using case management models. Case management approaches to HIV/AIDS care

are associated with fewer reported unmet needs and higher use of requisite medications (Katz et al., 2001).

Using a generalist model with common terminology to describe the core processes does not indicate uniformity or standardization of practice. Instead, it refers to the common problem-solving activities found in the helping process. The American Psychiatric Association (2000) has developed a set of commonly agreed-upon treatment guidelines to outline features of treatment from a psychiatric perspective. Some practice model differences relate to barriers to applications, interdisciplinary communication barriers, and unique problems found in AIDS work. For example, barriers to the application of the generalist model include the stigma of the clients, lack of familial supports, problems of client dementia, problems with discharge planning, conflicts over the advocacy process, and countertransference issues (Roberts et al., 1992).

Community-based care providers would more likely emphasize interorganizational or group relationship barriers especially among differing special populations (Indyk et al., 1993). For example, when working with women and children, the interactions tend to require services geared more to maternal and child health. When working with gay men, services linking with community-based support organizations become more critical. The dearth of these agencies and programs often further isolates persons, especially in rural, small town, and suburban areas. Other vulnerable persons who suffer from mental illness, drug use, racism, or cultural competency barriers may also be isolated.

Generalist practice using case management models has shown success in prevention of HIV infections ("HIV Prevention Through Case Management," 1993) and cost reductions (Pawlusiak and Hickman, 1966). With the growth of managed care in health service, roles may need to change to include advocacy with health delivery providers in such areas as documentation of need, the challenge to denials of care, coverage education, and mediating the linkage with advocacy groups. This may especially be true with the need for concomitant mental health care (Clifford, 1997). The high comorbidity of HIV and substance use and other mental health problems requires vigilance in data gathering in these areas. Where vulnerabilities are socially reinforced, generalist practice can address these social barriers, such as with gay men and lesbian women dealing with problems of coming out, heterosexism, and problems relating to community institutions (Garnet and D'Augelli, 1994). Practice in AIDS services needs to rely on the scientific problem-solving process in data gathering, as well as on the relationship-building process.

THE RELATIONSHIP PROCESS: ENGAGING CLIENT SYSTEMS IN SERVICES

The use of relationships in the helping process is at the heart of helping (Perlman, 1979). Though various practice models afford differing levels of emphasis on the relationship between the worker and the client, the generalist model assumption is that a positive working relationship is necessary to promote change in the client system. In an early "classic" examination of the relationship process, Biestek (1957) noted key features of the relationship as individualization, purposeful expression of feelings, controlled emotional involvements, acceptance, nonjudgmental attitudes, client self-determination, and confidentiality. These become the core of the basic relationship which is the obligation of the worker to establish and cultivate.

The core value inherent in all of social work practice is the belief in the dignity of every person. This becomes particularly challenged in the social contexts in which many persons become stigmatized and devalued, and when persons may engage in behaviors that are difficult to understand or may be potentially harmful to others. Acceptance and participation in services is connected to establishing a working relationship. The relationship-building process requires that the worker get to know the client system, whether individual, family, group, organization, or community. Involvement must be responsive to the individual, and not to stereotypes or images. This necessitates building a trusting relationship. Perlman (1979) lists the common elements necessary for building such a relationship: concern, commitment, acceptance, empathy, clear communication, genuineness, appropriate use of authority, and clarity of purpose.

Engaging the client system in the helping process requires trust and a willingness to commit to a relationship. Trust is afforded most readily when it has been earned and when it has not been severely breached in the past. The generalist model usually emphasizes the here and now, the present, but does not ignore past hurt. Judith Viorst (1986) provides examples of how persons who have experienced losses in their past can help shape their current willingness and capacity to develop trusting relationships.

An empowerment perspective in practice promotes viewing the relationship-building process as egalitarian and mutual (Mancoske and Hunzeker, 1990). All levels of service must be viewed from the prism of justice and equality. This includes developing a working relationship with the client system. When the focus is on problem solving, which the generalist model stresses, caution is required to avoid limiting perspectives to problems or deficits. This is done by examining strengths while assessing problems. Developing accurate empathy helps the service provider see the richness of the client system in its interactional whole.

Various barriers to the development of a working relationship occur and must be analyzed in the interactions between the worker and the client system. On an individual interpersonal level, these barriers are referred to as transference and countertransference. Transference is the conscious and unconscious feelings, wishes, fears, and defenses that influence the client's perceptions of the worker. Countertransference is the dynamic phenomenon that refers to the worker's feelings and defenses. In a psychodynamic model of practice, the emphasis is on unconscious aspects, whereas a generalist model emphasizes how these unconscious and conscious feelings influence current interpersonal dynamics. These feelings influence working relationships and their development and thus require attention when they impede trust and cooperation.

Cultural understandings and misunderstandings also shape the development of a working relationship. Many relationship barriers are rooted in the diversity of historical relationships and power imbalances among groups of people. The history of issues ranging from ethnocentricity to outright racial and ethnic hatred influences understandings between diverse groups. Solomon (1976) suggests that workers develop ethnic competencies: be aware of one's own ethnic limitations; be open to diversity; see all clients as an expression of cultural diversity; and acknowledge cultural integrity (noting actions that work in specific settings that may generate difficulties in other settings). Solomon (1976) expresses characteristics of a nonracist practitioner as able to perceive alternative explanations; able to see how clients perceive explanations; able to be warm and empathic; and able to confront distortions.

Gender diversity also requires cultural competency. The rise of fundamentalist religious forces that restrict women's roles in society and the feminization of poverty contribute to pervasive barriers to women's full development. Models of practice that focus on intrapersonal problems rather than the person in context reinforce pathologizing rather than the empowerment of all people. Promoting equality of relationships in generalist practice averts problems. Valentich (1986) discusses unequal relationships in which overdependence, in a self-fulfilling prophecy, is defined as a characteristic of women. Women with HIV face unique challenges based on gender roles and devaluations ascribed to these roles. They also face certain issues that may or may not be included in research or treatment studies. Some of these aspects relate to biological circumstances as well as gender order concerning reproductive and gynecologic issues. Working with females requires routine domestic violence screening (Klein, Birkhead, and Wright, 2000). Cohen and colleagues (2000) found support for the concern that a continuum of risk exists for women, for example, women who experienced sexual abuse as children had more experiences with domestic violence as adults, and higher HIV infection rates. These complex dynamic patterns impact relationship-building issues and may be central to the helping relationship processes. Such concerns as partner notification, prevention, testing, safety planning, and referrals become important concerns in areas that overlap between domestic violence and HIV. Women are at increased risk for delaying care, with serious health consequences because of responsibilities in caring for others, especially children in the home (Stein et al., 2000). Culturally competent practice in the relationship-building process implies that planned interventions directly address the range of special issues women face in light of caregiver burdens.

Sexual orientation also becomes a barrier to the development of a working relationship. Woodman (1989) summarizes some common themes that emerge in interpersonal interactions between workers and client systems: issues of loss (in the coming-out process, in dissonances between self-image and damaged roles, AIDS losses); anticipated losses (supports, employment discrimination, safety); personal identity threats (interpersonal devaluations, healthy paranoia, multiple oppressions), concerns about group identity (identity pressures, role models, power disparities between stigmatized subgroups), and relationship problems (lack of validation of relationships, family disruptions, discrimination, domestic violence, substance abuse). A cultural-competence model would necessitate not only familiarity with common forms of oppression but indications of trust would require evidence of commitment to change based on equity and mutuality of interests. Advocacy and social change activities are requisite practice skills for culturally competent practice with gay men and lesbian women.

Social service providers must confront their own traditions of racism, sexism, and homo-hatred before their commitment to social justice is accepted. Social workers work with a full spectrum of cultural and social diversity, and workers themselves are a reflection of this diversity. A social worker's personal outrage at discrimination against his- or herself does not uniformly assure the worker's cultural competency in working with other devalued populations. As an example of trying to see beyond one's own field of experience, Henry Louis Gates (1998) recently discussed a backlash among African Americans toward gays who claimed that their "victimization" experience is similar to the pain of racism. Effective generalist practice requires skills in engaging clients in a helping process—which is complicated by the level of one's cultural competence. Before trust can be established in working out relationship complexities, such as in areas of confidentiality and informed consent, the quality of the relationship must be established (Mancoske and Lindhorst, 1995). Understanding how discrimination impacts health outcomes is necessary in light of the overwhelming evidence of disparities in health outcomes for people who face discrimination. Williams and Rucker (2000) recently discussed how race, racism, and discrimination contribute to health disparities. They note that it is necessary to recognize that discrimination is routine and commonplace in society, and we need to recognize that this will be similarly prevalent in the delivery of medical care. Confronting this is necessary to address health disparities, and competency in doing so is requisite to bring about change.

AIDS and Cultural Competence in Relationship Building

The HIV epidemic in the United States continues to disproportionately impact vulnerable populations—men who have sex with men (whether gay identified or not), persons of color, and women. The first decade of the epidemic notably impacted gay urban males and required cultural competency in working among this population. Steady change has occurred as the epidemic moves into other populations, particularly among African Americans and Latinos, women, and gradually into non-urban areas (Lynch, Lloyd, and Fimbres, 1993). During the first decade of the epidemic many professionals lacked the cultural competency to deliver effective services. The connection between infection and risk behaviors should focus on these diversities rather than on vulnerabilities.

Service providers should understand and listen to those who are affected by HIV/AIDS—building a working relationship allows planning for help which is based on what the client systems perceive to be their needs. Needs vary among differing groups, localities, and persons. Problems vary in importance among individuals. Risks such as needle sharing, unprotected sex, or even psychological distress may or may not be disclosed, depending upon trust levels. This trust involves not only worker and client, but also general levels of trust among group members, family members, involved organizations, and communities. Thus it is necessary to work to promote trust at all levels to shape interactions. Recognizing diversity and working from the strength of communities via empowerment techniques promotes engaging hard-to-reach populations into helping situations (Dicks, 1994).

Many cultural features are unique as well as common among populations at risk for HIV infection populations. For example, Hispanic gay men or African-American gay men may have different at-risk behaviors, beliefs about risk, knowledge about safer practices, opposite-sex relations, or needle-sharing practices than do other gay male populations. Social supports, familial relations, or group identities may vary. Developing a working relationship may require skills in understanding the nuances of these diversities. Culturally competent practice with gay, lesbian, transgendered persons, or bisexuals requires understanding their oppression, their history, and their general and special characteristics (Holmes and Hodge, 1995).

Culturally specific practice models based on the exclusive features of the client are necessary (Goicoechea-Balbona, 1997). These include culturally specific descriptions of the target systems, the helping process, and the care delivery systems. The social worker requires sensitivity to language barriers and cultural variables such as the influences of family, religion, views of material resources necessary for help, verbal and nonverbal communication about sensitive and/or dreaded topics, and male/female conflicts. Differences exist and need to be addressed if communication is to support relationship building. Worldviews and communication styles influence this process.

The levels of interventions chosen should not be imposed by professional views of "what is needed or what helps" but negotiated in a complex interactional approach. For example, Mancoske and Lindhorst (1994) encourage the use of groups as an empowerment approach to self-help and mutual support among oppressed persons, but in some cultural contexts, this approach may be too indirect. Women's roles, including parenting, may become integral to helping needs. Unless these issues are respected, work becomes entangled in value conflicts with or without awareness. Wellness strategies must integrate women's cultural variables in role changes, health, and self-empowerment (Pizzi, 1992).

Promoting helpful changes within diverse populations requires communicating these changes to skeptical populations. Good intentions do not assure changes that will benefit everyone. Messages about HIV/AIDS to vulnerable populations come amid thunderous devaluations heard in the larger society. As the religious right builds media campaigns attacking the morality and decency of gay men and lesbian women, as the mechanisms for equal opportunity for African Americans and Hispanic Americans are attacked as "reverse discrimination," and as women's economic safety nets end as welfare as we know it ends, public health measures in communities are conflicted by intolerance and inequity. Efforts to build partnerships with communities are necessary, but they co-occur with efforts that promote disharmony and inequity. This hampers interpersonal interactions and makes relationship building complex and challenging. In generalist social work practice, this complexity becomes the challenge to effective practice.

The unique concerns of youth need special consideration if practice is to be culturally relevant. Many youths do not know their HIV status, and thus issues of access and education become particularly challenging. Many adults fail to inform youths, fail to provide services, and services may exclude youths because of various legal and policy concerns. On the other end of the age spectrum, culturally competent services must recognize the experiences and concerns exclusive to care provision for the elderly. For example, evidence shows that elderly American males tend to experience greater levels of depression in dealing with HIV disease (Heckman, 2000). Interventions for affect problems are integral to culturally appropriate service delivery.

Early care and treatment is cost effective and can dramatically improve the overall quality of life and health of PWAs (Presidential Advisory Council on HIV/AIDS, 2000). Participation of PWAs in decisions that affect their lives is essential for responding to the challenges of the HIV pandemic. Participation as full partners in the fight against HIV/AIDS builds upon the competencies and capacities of those most directly in harm's way.

THE DATA-GATHERING PROCESS

Initial Phase in the Helping Process

Engaging the client system in the helping process involves setting up the process to begin the work. Care providers should know the social history of the client system to begin the helping process. This requires gathering information to determine a useful intervention. The beginning process involves preparing the context for information sharing. How does the organization portray the helping stance?

From a generalist perspective, the data-gathering process includes an examination of all system levels and how they interact. For the purposes of description, the following text outlines the content of the typical social history. First, examine how these pieces interact in a total or holistic sense. This may involve greater emphasis on individual system levels but can also be based on organizational analysis or community practice initiatives. From an empowerment-based perspective, identify not only the usual sources of difficulties or problems, but also strengths.

Data-Gathering Issues in HIV Services

The course of HIV includes a wide array of psychosocial threats originating in the course of the disease itself and in the complexity of its treatments and social reactions to the illness. The disease presents distinctive stresses, such as the relative youthfulness of invididuals affected with a life-threatening or terminal illness and related issues of fear and loss. Determining the attainable quality of life requires skills and interventions that promote change and self-care. Clients need to understand what is being asked of them and have a stake in process outcomes. Questioning clients about sensitive areas such as sexual expression often causes misunderstanding of terminology, misrepresenting behaviors because of this uncertainty of terminology, and changing answers to fit limited understanding of questions (Binson and Catania, 1998).

Understanding the data is in part influenced by the individual's outlook and mental health. Optimism, hope, or relative fatalism influence which data are shared on an individual level. Overlapping issues influences the sharing of personal information. Clients who have chronic mental illness for example, may also engage in risky behaviors such as needle sharing or unprotected sexual activities. They may also have social risk factors, such as being homeless, financially destitute, jobless, and may be isolated from family and friends. These factors impact the capacity to be actively involved in risk reduction or health promotion activities. If the person is elderly, he or she may be less likely to be assessed on risk levels based on chronological development. Because of vulnerabilities concurrent with mental illness, for example, people's experience with violence or sexual abuse may not be examined.

Persons with substance abuse histories may have difficulty reporting at-risk behaviors. A close personal relationship enhances the accuracy of reporting risk compared with informal interviewing approaches (Morrison et al., 1995). Dementia, mood disorders, and anxiety disorders co-occur with HIV (Katz et al., 1996). Overlapping physical, cognitive, and emotional symptoms are common and may require more detailed social histories and various additional tests (Baumann, 1993). When comorbidity is suspected, then the data-gathering process indicates detailed examination of these areas.

Some clients face particular risks from numerous interacting forces. For example, women working in the sex industry tend to have risks enhanced by economic forces in addition to health risks, substance use (ATOD—alcohol, tobacco, and other drugs), a lack of social resources, homelessness, a history of physical or sexual abuse, social isolation, and perhaps adolescent status. Male sex workers may have many of the same HIV-risk variables (Snell, 1995). Some may be dealing with the challenges of sexual minority issues. One study of male-to-female transgendered persons found a 35 percent HIV infection rate across several urban sites (Clements-Nolle et al., 2001) and 65 percent of the study participants reported problems with depression. The attitudes of workers and the public messages about work with stigmatized and devalued persons all shape worker attitudes and worker and client interactions.

Do not make assumptions about age when gathering data. Elderly persons are potentially at risk, yet this risk is not always recognized by service providers (Gutheil and Chichin, 1991). Relying on assumptions of risk without taking a social history can lead to generalizations that overlook risk thus further harming clients (Briggs et al., 1995). Risk may include infection as well as burdens in caring for infected family members or partners.

Data gathering includes important family dimensions. With HIV services, family assessments also emphasize ongoing risk factors for spreading HIV infections, including risks within the family. Practice models that engage clients into care systems are necessary to promote public health. Culturally competent models of care address the range of cultural variables shaping decisions to seek care. Programs and services need to be modified based on evidence of which aspects promote care to families affected by HIV (Goicoechea-Balbona, 1998). Before families are labeled "difficult to reach," the context in which care is delivered needs to be examined.

Most health care is delivered by family members—sometimes families of choice or families of origin. Thus when gathering data, information on the family of choice as well as family of origin is necessary. "Reconnecting" of estranged family-of-origin members requires complex decisions about dangers as well as advantages. This decision is best made with the support of a worker but not by the worker. Family supports affect access to care, decisions about care utilization, and follow-up. The need to inform and involve families should be examined based on potential supports and other concerns. Families are generally deemed a source of support and assistance, although this is often not the case with HIV services. In some circumstances, persons may be estranged from families of origin because of drug use problems or sexual orientation separations, and families may or may not be an asset.

The course of HIV is influenced by the number of persons infected in the family. This raises questions about evaluating multiple losses, capacity for caring for self and others, making plans for the care of dependents, and perhaps about feelings of blame or guilt. It also requires examination of relative risk for infection of others, including children. Current improved treatments have reduced incidences of infants being infected by neonatal, birth, or breast-feeding routes. When children and parents are infected, grandparents in many families becomes a potential source of care (Joslin and Brouard, 1995). Care boundaries move beyond health delivery into other social service and child welfare delivery systems, including services targeting the needs of the elderly. Services incorporating family systems often cross boundaries reflecting the needs of the child, the parent, the grandparent, and those institutions with which each interact. The families also face economic, social, emotional, and psychological threats. These internal and social stresses combine to influence the overall mental health and social functioning of the families (Roth, Siegel, and Black, 1994). Thus, data gathering includes various family dimensions and must include evidence of resiliency and strength to determine risk levels and coping capacities. The ecomap suggested by Hartman and Laird (1983) is a tool to gather evidence of the social network supports and strengths families have to offer and to understand those experiences in their environmental contexts.

Gathering data on the group influences in HIV care is vital. In some cases, persons may have a network of friends who become a family of choice replacing biological families. In other cases, such as among many adolescents, group influences become a strong developmental phenomenon indicating sources of support and strength. Assessing group influences requires data gathering to determine strengths and weaknesses. Skill levels vary between males and females, and between different ethnic groups of adolescents, but skill building has shown to be effective in risk reduction (Blumberg et al., 1997). Social distress such as homelessness or intrafamilial distress such as child abuse or sexual abuse exacerbates HIV risk.

Service providers should gather data on the organizations interacting with PWAs. These may be the organizations that workers represent as well as other providers of care. Agencies may make decisions about whom is to be served based on financial, community, or best practices decisions. They may have to choose between serving many or serving a few who show the most likelihood of improvement. Decisions may be based on sound outcome information or on prejudice.

As pressure for accountability mounts, agencies may avoid providing care to those most at risk or the most vulnerable, seeking to first work with the more readily treatable. Those with substance abuse problems require difficult work and some agencies are placing them last in line for care (Sorensen and Miller, 1996).

Some organizations, such as prisons, will require ongoing pressure to provide humane and adequate care and treatment. This population is at particular risk and requires much more attention than it receives, in part because of organizational constraints on service delivery as well as interorganizational conflicts about philosophy and service delivery. Persons being released from the criminal justice system pose challenges and public health is jeopardized by neglect of this population. Aggressive outreach is essential in connecting the hard-to-reach and vulnerable with services. Fund limitations may cause organizations to have difficulty achieving outreach objectives. In addition, organizations may prefer to work with "willing" clients and find reasons why outreach is not achievable. The National Institutes on Drug Abuse (2000) examined best practices in outreach for "out-of-treatment" substance users and suggest ways to provide successful outreach such as the following:

- start outreach programs early;
- emphasize risk reduction;
- provide multiple sites for service delivery;
- target those already infected;
- focus on couples;
- provide interventions in the natural environments;
- personalize interventions;
- demonstrate cultural sensitivity and cultural competency;
- provide access to clean needles and injection equipment;
- focus on sexual transmission risk reduction;
- sustain HIV interventions over time; and
- promote cost effectiveness of community-based efforts.

Community outreach efforts need to be integrated into family, organization, and community dynamics to provide effective behavioral change.

Gathering data at the organizational level may include measuring how well adapted the organization is in integrating "best practices" or "evidence-based care" into its service delivery. Clients need successful treatments implemented into service delivery. Kelly and colleagues (2000) describe various models with strategies for improving organizational responsiveness to innovations in care delivery and adaptation of best practices.

The complexity of PWAs' needs brings various organizations together in services for families, and these interactions may require interventions in dealing with interdisciplinary and interorganizational concerns. Organizations in rural areas may develop new resources based on developing community and local government support (Topping, Hartwig, and Cecil, 1997). Assessing the capacities of communities to provide care delivery defines the data-collection process. Ryan White legislation established councils which have principal responsibility for promoting needs assessments and planning for HIV/AIDS services. Many persons who are receiving treatment are assessed for their full range of needs. Thus, when gathering data on a client system, data collected in community-based needs assessments become core to the process.

In rural areas, community variables generally include barriers such as social and geographic isolation. PWAs often live far from medical care and have transportation and child care barriers. Workers in rural areas require generalist skills given the wide range of services a provider is required to deliver and the lack of specialty care available even when indicated (Lishner et al., 1996).

Case Example

LaTonya, a twenty-six-year-old African-American woman, has come to your agency requesting help after finding out that she is HIV positive. She is pregnant and was tested by her OB-GYN in a routine screening. LaTonya was shocked to find out she was HIV positive. She thinks she became infected by a former boyfriend who injected drugs. She does not know where he is and her current boyfriend for the past three years does not know she is infected. They usually use condoms but she started on birth control pills which she does not take regularly. She is worried that her two children (ages five and two) might also be infected. She has been working in a real estate office full time but does not have health insurance. She is looking for a better job that will offer health insurance. No one knows of her infection, including her mother with whom she is very close. Her mother has high blood pressure and LaTonya worries about her mother's health. She is afraid to have the baby because of the risk to the baby's health. She has been feeling "run down" the past few months—has fevers, colds, and frequent vaginal infections. She has seen medical providers but has not spoken with an HIV specialist. She appears angry, withdrawn, and she says she cries frequently when she is alone.

The Biopsychosocial Data

This case addresses the general questions asked—a social history. It does not address how or when the information is to be obtained. This is a process contingent upon characteristics of the relationship process and the persons, place, and context involved. If particular problems are indicated, more explicit levels of data are needed. Otherwise, a general review of problems and strengths are examined in order to plan for interventions (Mancoske and Hunzeker, 1990). As the relationship progresses, further biopsychosocial information is obtained and clarified. Following is an example of some of the data generally gathered in this process beyond the basic agency eligibility criteria and the presenting problem:

Physical

- *physical development:* developmental history; normal and exceptional life-span development
- *health:* individual health history (medications, illnesses, hospitalizations, symptoms); births; family health history (family of origin and family of choice, genogram)
- *physical environment:* safety; nutrition; space; contaminants; shelter; resources; neighborhood
- *influential patterns:* smoking; alcohol; other drugs; injection of drugs; stress; accident risks
- *sexual history:* experiences; satisfaction; orientation; disease; pregnancy; partner history; abuse

Psychological

- *psychosocial development:* developmental milestones; maturity; commitments; relationship history
- *cognition:* thinking; capacities; limitations; performance; group identities; education
- *behaviors:* risk patterns; relationships; personality disorders; defenses

- *emotions:* feelings; mood; suicide risk
- *aspirations:* hopes; dreams; spiritual development; religiosity; experiences with devaluation
- *mental health:* coping strategies; mental status; interpersonal skills; mental illnesses or personality disorders; adaptiveness

Social

- *Interactions:* between individual and groups; family; organizations; communities; roles; institutional norms and involvements; neighborhoods; ecomap of person in environment interactions (Hartman and Laird, 1983)
- *service eligibility status:* e.g., income; legal status; agency mission
- *resources:* finances; employment and work history; work conditions; educational opportunities; insurance; social supports; status, power, and influence
- *cultural resources:* origins; identities; supports; beliefs; traditions; religions; experiences with racism; language; cultural fit
- *families:* see also Hartman and Laird, 1983, for model for analysis; interactions with other systems; generational issues; internal dynamics
- *risks:* domestic violence; community violence; experiences with discrimination
- *cultural resources and connections:* church; civic; cultural stories/roles; assimilation and diversity; beliefs and attitudes; religious and spiritual beliefs

This biopsychosocial model is used as a general data-gathering process. The model facilitates organization of useful data in developing a working assessment and planning with clients for interventions. This list is not exclusive of other data, nor exhaustive of reasonable domains. The model affords opportunities to identify potential barriers to functioning, strengths and supports, and leads to more in-depth analysis in areas which may be indicative of further exploration. The model discourages focus on disease or pathology, encourages strengths and aspirations, and emphasizes interactions at all system levels.

ASSESSMENT

Assessments are often called by various names in the social work practice literature: social diagnosis or diagnosis, case studies, psychosocial diagnosis. The generalist model emphasizes interactions between social systems and focuses upon strength and empowerment as well as identifying problems or deficits. The assessment terminology fits the model better than diagnosis, which implies more focus on identification of specific disorders or psychopathological processes. However, social workers both assess problems and diagnose mental health problems and substance abuse problems by tradition and in many states by license laws.

With the data-gathering process built upon the strength of the relationship-building process, a professional opinion is indicated regarding the worker's view of the problems. This opinion should be mutually arrived at by cooperation between the worker and client. In some circumstances, workers may have assessments of problems that diverge from the opinions of the clients. However, from an empowerment perspective, the process of reaching an assessment is mutual.

The social work assessment in a generalist model identifies the focus of the problem with which a contract for services is to be planned and established. At times, a "triage" issue requires an assessment focus. For example, if the client is a danger to self or to others, or if the client is involved in child abuse or neglect, this cannot be left out of the assessment. No matter which problems the client may wish to focus upon, some problems, by law and by ethical code, require the primary focus of the worker. Mandatory reporting and the duty to warn are essential.

Assessments in HIV/AIDS Services

A clear delineation of a particular problem (or problems) mutually agreed upon by worker and client to be the focus of work together is essential to good assessments. The problems need to be stated in measurable terms and the goals of interventions need to be identifiable. The problems can occur at any system level—individual, family, group, organization, or community—in which evidence exists that interventions are effective. How HIV/AIDS diminishes the quality of life of the client system becomes the general overall goal of establishing a working contract to address specific problems.

Given the existential challenges a person with life-threatening or terminal illness faces, focus for some should begin with issues on the individual level that deal with intrapersonal issues. This may be spiritual or life review type foci. Development of better interpersonal strengths may be needed, such as skills in intimacy-building care strategies which help provide meaning and support to enhance well-being (Kendall, 1996). The focus may be on psychoeducational aspects of coping with HIV disease, such as management of symptoms, pain, medications, or support resources essential to practical adaptation to the sick role. This process requires an activist role in learning about treatment options, alternative treatments, and it requires an efficacious self-advocacy in securing care in a health care system that is highly specialized and bureaucratized. It may require care planning in the event of a particular health crisis, such as dimentia, which limits one's ability to make such health care decisions as planning wills, indicating advanced directives, or designating medical power of attorney. This may also require dealing with affective disorders that co-occur with various disease manifestations and treatment regimens.

Some PWAs also live with mental illness. The incidence of mental illness co-occurring with substance abuse among PWAs is especially high—about seventeen times higher than in the general population (HIV/AIDS Bureau, 2000, p. 5). Substance abuse and addiction compromise the ability of individuals to secure quality care and to stay in care. The HIV/AIDS Bureau (2000) report indicates also that without substance abuse treatment, HIV treatment has almost no chance for success. In a study of Medicaid beneficiaries in one state, it was found that persons with substance use disorders were more likely to have problems with serious mental illness (Walkup, Crystal, and Sambamoorthi, 1999). This population's mental health is often overlooked in practice because of concerns with the substance use disorders and the HIV. These multiple-diagnosed concerns require more complex treatments, although treatment effectiveness is improving in the separate areas. Rosenberg and colleagues (2001) note over a dozen research studies examining the elevated rates of HIV infections among persons with severe mental illness. When persons experience problems with severe mental illness as well as general affective disorders co-occurring with HIV, concerns with prevention and responsible sexual relations become more complicated as well.

HIV often manifests as a series of crises, which when interacting with other vulnerabilities and depending upon one's strengths, resources, and supports, may lead to suicide risk. Persons with life-threatening illness or terminal illness are at enhanced risk for suicide—with HIV, the risk may well be higher for a variety of reasons (Mancoske et al., 1995). Suicide risk appears to be associated with the stress experienced by gay men (Remafedi et al., 1998). As in all assessments, triage issues are initially ruled out and constantly reviewed and reassessed. Suicide risk needs renewed focus as work progresses (Maris et al., 1992), especially during particularly vulnerable periods associated with HIV, such as initial diagnosis or during terminal phases. This is a complicated area of concern, and may lead to a discussion of rational suicide and self-deliverance. However, the beginning point of this discussion and major focus is on prevention of suicide until all other risks are ruled out or clarified.

Because some persons do not respond well to treatments, or have serious and persistent problems with associated illnesses, despair may need to be a focus of risk assessment. Since affective symptoms co-occur with dementia, both need to be evaluated, and both may indicate different intervention planning. Recognizing and investigating neuropsychiatric as well as psychological manifestations of dementia are important. This should be an interdisciplinary process so that the full range of risk markers is examined—physical, psychological, and social. Accurate appraisal does not guarantee safety (Motto, 1991) but it does promote well-being. Some typical cognitive markers for workers to note include changes in intelligence, attention span, speed in thinking, memory, abstraction, language, visual perception, construct thinking, motor abilities, and mental status (Butters et al., 1990).

Some persons may be doing well physically with medical treatments but may be suffering psychologically with multiple losses or survivors' guilt. They may be facing decisions about work, disability planning, insurance coverage, or finances. Many persons with serious illness have severe psychological distress which is responsive to medical and psychosocial interventions. As rates of infection among women increase, some family issues such as permanency planning, disclosure issues, guilt over prior behaviors, and/or caring for ill children or partners may also multiply (National Abandoned Infants Resource Center, 2002). Most caregiving is provided by women, and this burden is not absolved when women assume illness roles.

Given the grief, shock, sadness, anxiety, stress, and related aspects of HIV disease for individuals and their support networks, family assessments are essential, and workers need to involve families with maintaining and enhancing the integrity and supportiveness of the family. Demoralization can be induced by complications of the illnesses, the attendant psychological distress, and social consequences such as loss of income, jobs, or permanent living arrangements. All interact in a synergistic manner thus creating health peril. Suggested ways of promoting support include encouraging open communication, educating about AIDS illness, developing self-protection, and maintaining outside interests and supports (Lippmann, James, and Frierson, 1993). Advocacy regarding securing basic support services is a core intervention necessity. Issues found in the data-gathering process need to be considered in all levels of assessment, such as the impact of substance abuse on multiple system levels. Self-medicating via use of alcohol may induce complications of dysphoric mood or in interactive processes, dysphoric mood may trigger relapse.

Co-occurring mental illnesses may be exacerbated by physical health problems or by attendant stressors (Bartlett, 2001). Left untreated, they may intensify psychosocial distress or impair health outcomes. Persons with depression are less likely to comply with medical recommendations. Bartlett (2001) identifies a range of overlapping issues in treating HIV medical conditions conjointly with mental disorders. Some physical problems, such as strokes, may generate depressive symptoms. HIV is not a causal factor in schizophrenic disorders, but persons with schizophrenia may exhibit impaired judgment about HIV risk factors. Premorbid anxiety disorders complicate treatments, and the usual concerns about comedicating and addictive potentials are accompanying risks. Working with persons with comorbid psychiatric disorders requires interdisciplinary practice in which the psychiatrist often becomes an important provider of specialized services following particular treatment guidelines that overlap the functions of care provision by other providers. Coordination of care requires that team decisions recognize the specialty care guidelines (American Psychiatric Association, 2000) and from an empowerment perspective, that the person living with HIV be fully informed and involved in all care decisions.

Community-based needs assessments involve data-gathering and determinations that are based on a wide range of needs. A case management approach is indicated to address the multiple system levels of need. In case management models of care delivery, when the problems are identified, plans for interventions are developed. Interventions may cut across all system levels, though a narrower range is often the focus.

INTERVENTIONS

Interventions in generalist practice address the problems noted in the data-gathering process and which are mutually agreed upon by worker and client as the focus of the assessment. The interventions address problems at any system level and quite often involve multiple system levels. Generally, concerns are prioritized and those most pressing become the main focus. Some primary problems include substance abuse, family violence, or intention to harm others. Such overriding issues must be addressed, or others are less likely to be resolved. It is difficult to establish a working contract with clients when the worker's assessments diverge from the client's. Unless a triage situation necessitates immediate action, such as with child abuse or neglect, or threats to harm oneself or others, workers may agree to focus on a problem that the client identifies as the priority and not directly address the primary issue as identified by the social worker—at least for a temporary time until evaluations of success can be assessed and until the relationship is strengthened.

Interventions generally employ generic tactics in the helping process. The tactics address various levels of practice, from the organizational change, community-organizing and policy-changing tactics common to macropractice to counseling techniques common to individual-level interventions. Northen (1994) identifies common psychosocial techniques used: relationship building, structuring, exploration, confrontation, ventilation, instilling hope, clarification, education and advice giving, and facilitating interactions. Empowerment-focused models stress collaborating, utilizing small groups, consciousness raising, teaching skills, using mutual aid, and mobilizing resources (Gutierrez, 1989).

Specific problems must be targeted and goals established that allow measurable outcomes to be determined. The working contract with the client system needs to clearly establish roles, responsibilities, and how outcomes are to be evaluated. Be explicit for clarification purposes as well as to motivate participation. Other practice models rely more on insight development and may not emphasize the collaboration and mutuality of empowerment-based generalist practice (Mancoske and Hunzeker, 1990). In addition, considerations of special populations and cultural competence may not be emphasized in the intervention approach. The use of authority in generalist practice is more egalitarian and mutual, and this is only superceded in triage issues, e.g., risk for suicide or harming others. Resistance is viewed as occuring less at an unconscious level (although this does have some influence on practice), but more at a conscious level. Practice focuses on the here and now and the core of relationship development is to instill trust, hope, and a sense that change can occur, and thus resistence is directly handled in the relationship-building process. Some work may be done at the "unconscious level" (Cohler and Galatzer-Levy, 2000), though this is generally not the focus of work. Interventions in various settings influenced by managed care service environments encourage the use of brief interventions and crisis interventions.

Interventions in HIV/AIDS Services

Interventions target the system level where change is directed. At the individual level, the complexity of new treatments in the medical arena often dictates that some attention be focused upon decision making and adherence to complicated treatment regimens. Depression associated with HIV/AIDS is a treatable disorder. Interventions not only include medical care and medications, but a combined focus on positive outlooks, stress management, planning for wellness, and dealing with grief (National Institute of Mental Health [NIMH], 2002). Persons who receive optimal medical care may not receive appropriate or adequate mental health care.

Education about pathways of the illness may be a focus, and skills in coping, adapting, and managing the illness may be part of a psychosocial analogue to other treatments. Interventions such as stress management and coping strategies improve quality of life in various dimensions (Lutgendorf et al., 1994). Problems identified should become part of the planned interventions to improve health and social functioning. For example, if a person is experiencing depression, it should not be viewed as simply "understandable," but as a focus of intervention. Research has linked depression with the progression of HIV disease (Ickovics, 2001) and thus the impetus is for effective interventions. Interdisciplinary practice requires that roles be clarified and client needs be the focus of the interventions—the client may of course be individuals, organizations, neighborhoods, or communities.

When particular problems are identified, the research on intervention effectiveness should be examined. For example, in HIV services, problems of mood disorders are treatable using standard psychotherapeutic techniques along with medications (Markowitz et al., 1998). In an editorial in *The Washington Post,* drug czar Barry McCaffrey (1998) also described recent studies by the NIMH which indicated that drug abuse treatment programs of many types (inpatient, outpatient, self-help) are all effective in reducing drug use, crime, and recidivism. Although in Washington, DC, for example, only 10 percent of persons seeking treatment can readily access substance abuse treatment. Social workers in HIV services and in mental health services provide considerable care to those with substance abuse issues given the high comorbidity in these fields. Substance abuse treatment is effective in prevention of further HIV infections according to a study reported by Metzger, Navaline, and Woody (1998). Thus, proven effective interventions need to be part of the intervention planning. Many of the interventions are transferrable—addressing problems in one area to improve functioning has a synergistic effect on the quality of life in other interactional areas.

Interventions need to address the spectrum of HIV—from primary prevention, testing, early infection, AIDS diagnosis, experiences with serious illnesses, harm reduction to end-stage illnesses (Shernoff, 1998). These issues may need to be addressed during early stages of denial and into planned interventions that promote the person's capacities for making choices about one's own health and well-being. Undoing health disparities requires vigilance in addressing disparate outcomes for the poor and for minorities. African-Americans and Hispanic persons are less likely to be involved in experimental treatments, which contributes to disparities (Cunningham, 2002).

When an intervention plan addresses comorbidity of HIV and substance abuse, services must be integrated to be most effective (Center for Substance Abuse Treatment [CSAT], 2000). Many challenges to integrating HIV and substance abuse care exist—including differences in priorities and treatment philosophies, funding sources, and provider training. The CSAT report recommends working toward a shared treatment philosophy, a strong case management model, the delivery of core social services, training across HIV and substance abuse, and shared eligibility determinations. The CSAT report goes on to address the importance of cultural competency issues which highlight the particular needs of the special populations served and planned interventions specific to the care activities.

Interventions at the individual level have considerable impact on the family level and thus most social work care plans incorporate family issues into strategies. Family systems are profoundly impacted by life-threatening illness and must be evaluated for problems and as resources in care provision (Sholevar and Perkel, 1990). After recognizing the cautions as noted earlier regarding families, generally families are involved in care. Listen first to the voice of the individual, then provide education to partners/spouses, children, parents, and grandparents. Issues of mental health, health care, substance abuse, role changes, needs of families, and child care interact with the planned interventions, whether they are directly or indirectly addressed. How various cultural and ethnic group families understand and experience the challenges of HIV shapes how the individuals experience the disease and care during the disease. Interventions on behalf of individuals may be provided to families, extended families, or to neighborhoods through education, support, or outreach thus involving multiple system levels into the care of individuals. Education and health promotion in African-American communities require that issues of sexual orientation and/or drug-using behaviors and how they interact among various community leaders should become a focus (Icard et al., 1992).

Social supports make a difference in improved health outcomes and families traditionally provide the core of social supports for persons with illnesses and disabilities (Rolland, 1994). There are unique barriers to care found in HIV services, such as stigma and family alienation because of issues of sexual orientation or drug use. Families can be barriers to care rather than social support assets. Families may in fact become a major source of tension or stress. These supports are influenced by projections of blame, attitudes about obligation, fears of infection, attitudes toward homosexuality or drug use, shared family stigma, and family stability (McDonell, Abell, and Miller, 1991).

Interventions with families may be indicated to deal with these issues. Support issues for concrete service needs may require advocacy skills. Families may require information and referral as well as specific services to address their needs before they are able to continue sharing in care activities. When discussing families, we recognize that some are alternative families—including gay and lesbian families and their children. Grandparents or other relatives who are informally providing care can be included as are foster families.

From an empowerment perspective, group work is generally a preferable option for service provision because of its emphasis on egalitarianism and mutual support. For some populations, such as adolescents who turn to peers for guidance, and for gay men and lesbians who often must develop peer supports in the face of hostile social environments, groups are important interventions. When family-of-origin hostility or rigidity characterize social networks, expanding involvements by families of choice or by groups may be a viable option for promotion of care. In some cultural communities, in which opinions are hostile to issues of gay culture and language or intergenerational beliefs add to isolation, small support groups can supplant family estrangement or hostility. Common features may unite persons into mutual aid when other resources may not be as uniting, such as in groups for HIV-negative gay men (Koetting, 1996).

Spirig (1998) reviewed the literature on support groups for people living with HIV/AIDS and noted that these support groups reduce stress, improve coping, and provide needed social supports. Support groups have worked well in other health problem areas, such as for persons living with breast cancer. Their applications have been developed in various and innovative areas, such as upon initial diagnosis (Samarel, Fawcett, and Tulman, 1997), with advanced cancer (Greenstein and Breitbart, 2000), and even with online support groups for persons in maintenance phases (Page et al., 2000). Reports include such benefits as symptom decrease, functional status improvement, improved quality of life, reduced emotional distress, and a sense of finding meaning in life.

Specificity about outcome objectives is essential to determining the success of group outcomes. Success can involve both individual improvements in psychosocial functioning (DiPasquale, 1990) or changes in the group process itself. The focus may be on changing attitudes, knowledge, or risky behaviors via family member support groups. Groups may be developed to address unique needs of PWAs, such as women's support groups which focus on concrete resource development for children's needs, to resolve individual problems such as substance abuse, or to resolve domestic violence issues. In a review of the literature examining the effectiveness of HIV counseling in prevention of HIV, Weinhardt and colleagues (1999) summarize findings which indicate that counseling does not appear to provide primary prevention for infections, although it has shown to be effective in secondary infection preventions. Thus, using evaluations can help focus counseling activities to maximize potential, as well as to effectively channel psychosocial and financial resources.

Interventions at the macro level, such as organizations and communities, also are important options to address the specific problems of PWAs. Many barriers to care can be addressed by social workers at the organizational level, such as problems with lack of care coordination, conflicting policies between care organizations, barriers to access concerning concrete needs or service eligibility issues, or connecting people to existing care. For these reasons, case management systems initially looked appealing to Ryan White-funded care systems. At times, service needs are defined from the bottom up, such as the advocacy efforts to establish needle exchange programs in various at-risk communities. The resistance often does not originate with the local communities as much as from external forces that have political agendas distinct and in conflict with public health measures. Needle exchange programs offer evidence of effectiveness without increasing drug risk (Heimer, 1998). Other mutual-aid-type organizations developing in various communities include gay and lesbian health clinics found in about thirteen urban areas. Resources in rural areas are few but are emerging. Care and services may be provided by specialized AIDS services organizations or integrated into existing service delivery systems. Each community must be assessed for its resources and social workers' information and referrals become important sources of community development.

Generalist practice often addresses problems at multiple system levels. An example of this is found in recommendations of the United Nations AIDS Program (2002) in addressing problems of the elderly living with HIV. Recommendations include multiple system level interventions for the elderly such as: efforts to reduce stigma; integrating HIV services into elderly health care; provider training; specific research addressing the elderly with HIV; and services driven by elderly involvement. Services at the multiple systems level allows for a broad array of practice interventions.

Most HIV/AIDS services are not directly funded in federal HIV/AIDS services program, however most financial support comes through Medicaid and Medicare. This of course includes from state and local matching funds. At the local level, money comes from both public and private sources. Hence, developing coordinated and planned care delivery systems requires working with diverse planning and capital resources.

EVALUATION OF SERVICES

In applying the scientific model to practice using the generalist model, systematic examination of service effectiveness is required. This is not only a necessity of the scientific process, but a core element of the helping process which allows service providers to receive feedback on how well service planning and interventions are working.

A variety of approaches exist to analyze evidence of service effectiveness. Some seem to offer more guidance on how overall services affect client system changes such as using comparison designs or program evaluations. Another approach is to examine how particular interventions work with particular individuals using a single-case design approach. No methodology is without limitations, and each offers some evidence of effectiveness. The following section offers examples of how various types of design inform practice. Practitioners need to make decisions about care based on supporting evidence for their plans found in the literature and provide interventions that offer evidence of effectiveness.

HIV/AIDS Service Effectiveness

One example of evidence in practice that helps control the spread of HIV infections is to connect substance abusers with competent treatment. Research has shown that drug abuse treatment is one of the best ways to control the spread of HIV and its health consequences (Hanson, 2002). Hanson goes on to note that, unfortunately, over 85 percent of chronic drug abusers are not in treatment. The challenge is to increase access to effective services. The National Institutes on Drug Abuse (NIDA, 2002) summarizes principles of HIV prevention that have produced positive results among substance abusers:

- reduction of HIV is achievable;
- early intervention is effective;
- effectiveness requires comprehensive services;
- prevention involves whole communities assessing problems and evaluating effectiveness;
- services need to be neighborhood-based with responsive service hours;
- services need to involve those already infected and their social networks (sex partners, families, etc.);
- services need to be individualized, culturally competent, respectful of diversity, and sustained over time;
- access to clean needles supports prevention;
- risk reduction alone is less efficient than when combined with more traditional counseling and behavioral change approaches; and
- prevention is cost effective.

An example of using research findings to inform practice is the reported research on outcomes of substance abuse treatment programs funded by the Substance Abuse and Mental Health Services Administration (1998). This large-scale survey of persons in substance abuse treatment confirms that drug abuse and criminal behavior are reduced following inpatient, outpatient, and residential treatment for drug abuse. The overall reduction in drug use was 21 percent for all drugs, the highest reduction being for cocaine use. The reduction was larger for females and lower for adolescents. Those remaining in treatment the longest had the highest success rates. Other findings indicated that criminal activities were reduced, physical abuse and suicide attempts declined, parenting factors showed improvement, and housing stability improved. This large-scale study validates earlier studies indicating similar findings. Many of these studies were specific to HIV and substance abuse (Needle, Coyle, and Normand, 1998). The cost-benefit findings urge additional funding for drug treatment programs. Even high-risk women with substance abuse problems show cost-benefit reduction in HIV risk by counseling programs (Owens, Brandeauu, and Sox, 1998). Methadone maintenance treatment programs, for example, have reduced HIV costs, and provide benefits in the public health and social arena as well (Zaric, Barnett, and Brandeau, 2000). Prevention programs also are demonstrably effective with a variety of at-risk populations as reported by the CDC's HIV/AIDS Prevention Research Synthesis Project (CDC, 1999).

An example of using evidence-based interventions in practice is the effectiveness of using support groups in work with PWAs. Spirig (1998) reviewed the literature and notes that various studies indicate the benefits of this approach. However, further large-scale research studies and intervention trials would be valuable. Many studies of support groups in other settings and with other diagnoses exist, and there are reasonable assumptions of transferability to work in HIV/AIDS care. Spiegel et al. (1989) report on studies with control populations and experimental interventions and with long-term follow-up showing the sound success of psychosocial treatments provided by support groups, including an impact on improving long-term survival for breast cancer. In another empirical study of persons with cancer, support groups showed similar successes in emotional health and symptom reduction (Magen and Glajchen, 1999). In further research on the effectiveness of support groups for women with breast cancer, Gore-Felton and Spiegel (1999) report on two decades of research showing evidence in reducing mood disturbance, improving quality of life, enhancing psychological functioning, and increasing survival time. Leserman (1999) reports that developing social supports via treatment groups is a critical health care objective to improve survival and slow the progression of HIV disease. Leserman (2000) further reports that denial and stress speed the progression of HIV disease. Evidence-based practice certainly indicates that support group interventions are essential components of successful HIV care.

Another area of critical importance to HIV services is compliance with medications. The literature shows that even the more difficult-to-reach clients can show improvement with services promoting adherence and problem solving. Some of the interventions are related to medical technology and monitoring and some relate to education on benefits and risks (Hecht, 1998). Compliance is such a critical issue that it should be part of the general data-gathering process. This does not imply that PWAs be induced to comply with medications, only that they make informed decisions, and that treatment should include adequate assessments of barriers to adherence. Noncompliance is associated with depression and psychological distress (Singh et al., 1996) and thus interacts with the holistic and interdisciplinary intervention plan.

Support for enabling PWAs to make health care decisions is at the heart of the empowerment-based generalist model. When persons see benefits, they are more likely to cooperate. Research from a variety of studies indicates that nearly one-third of medical procedures performed in this country are of questionable health benefit relative to their risk (McGlynn and Brook, 1996). Informing practice requires viewing problems at more than one system level.

Program evaluations also offer social workers knowledge of whether services are effective by examining organizational and community-level data. For example, a study of one Ryan White Planning Council (San Francisco) using a program evaluation approach to multiple providers found that the services were reaching intended populations, that improvements were being evidenced, and that unmet needs called for additional services (Marx et al., 1997). The Ryan White CARE Act does not fund evaluations, though it assumes that responsible administrative agents are producing program evaluations. Some evidence of these concerns are noted in conference presentations.

Another way that the scientific process in helping models can offer evidence of effectiveness is if single-case designs are implemented in the helping process and data are used to systematically monitor performance and outcomes. This means that individual intervention plans are systematically monitored by the worker and client system to determine changes by predesigned measures used before, during, and following interventions. Some degree of experimental change is generally employed. Outcome standards are applied that either directly or indirectly measure desired outcomes. Replications are usually used. An example of this model for receiving input into the effectiveness of interventions is found in a description of a single system design using several measures (Orgnero and Rodway, 1991).

Evaluations are always necessary to examine the consequences of interventions. Sometimes unintended consequences have immediate bearing on service outcomes and effectiveness. Ironically, as HIV treatments become more effective, and as medical interventions become more successful, they may impede social and psychosocial interventions. For example, as HIV becomes more of a chronic disease than a uniformly fatal illness, benefits such as Social Security and disability may become more complex and difficult to secure. Legal protections may be diminished as medical interventions become more successful. Hence, adherence problems may well have further damaging consequences. As federal spending continues to increase in HIV services, demands for accountability emanate not only from the funding sources, but from the professionals delivering the range of psychosocial and medical interventions. As "faith-based providers" take on greater service roles, it will be interesting to note how continuous quality improvement issues will be implemented and promoted in service delivery. This may also further complicate what is known about sexual minorities experiencing HIV (Battle and Bennett, 2000). Sexual minority persons of color have traditionally been overlooked in service delivery needs, and changing delivery models may enhance concerns of some as well as limit them for others.

Unintended consequences of interventions may also have to deal with iatrogenic problems brought about by medication errors. A trend in increased dispensing errors is evident as interventions become more complex and more medications enter the treatment market (Purdy, 2000). Purdy notes that these errors are common—and preventable. Various types of errors are described: prescribing the wrong drugs, doses, frequency, and other problems such as drug/drug or food/drug interactions. Evaluations of practice must include wide ranges of interventions: including the psychosocial issues and their interactions with medical interventions.

THE TERMINATION PROCESS

Termination is the ending phase of the helping process. Termination begins with a discussion of engaging client systems into the helping process; gathering data necessary to understand the problems and strengths of the client systems; an assessment of the key problems and strengths which will be the focus of the helping process; a plan for interventions that addresses the mutually agreed upon problems; a plan for evaluation that provides evidence of effectiveness of the interventions in the working process; and when the objectives have been met, the process of ending ensues.

Endings are integral to the problem-solving process for various reasons. They are a part of the chronological phases of helping. Recognize that in human relationships, endings may be difficult for some to handle, and they may symbolize other issues of loss which bring pain. Poorly handled endings may perhaps set persons back to prior levels of functioning and thus may undo progress achieved in the intervention process. Also, endings need to reinforce the positive aspects of change as well as answer questions about future helping resources, and thus various requisites are needed to accomplish endings. Finally, it is a chance to ritualize the ending in ways that affirm values gained in the helping process, by both the client system and the worker.

One element of the termination process is to evaluate the potential risks and harm of endings. If clients are particularly vulnerable because of recent or repeat losses, then their capacity and strengths, the potentials of their support networks, and their trust in themselves become part of the ending assessments. When goals are accomplished, the process of ending is part of the overall helping process. Endings should be discussed when work commences and reviewed for relevancy as the work phases are accomplished.

HIV/AIDS and the Termination Process

The crises of AIDS are many, and none more omnipresent than the existential challenges posed by the epidemic. Some good may come from crisis. The Chinese characters for the word "crisis" are "risk" and "opportunity." It may be a time for a deepening spirituality, a firm commitment to relationships, a time when expressions of love are least hampered by the mundane. Experienced workers who have addressed some of these questions in their personal lives may be more responsive to clients searching for such growth. Confronting one's own mortality affects not only the PWA but also those within their intimate network. Services must not only address issues of loss and endings with the entire client system, but recognize the diverse ways people cope with these issues. The kinds and amount of loss and whether persons anticipating losses are dealing with their own mortality because of also being HIV infected or for other reasons, shape the experiences (Chidwick and Borrill, 1996). Different responses to loss are likely—from rapid acceptance to violently negative feelings.

These are influenced by the stages of the disease as well as the personal and social strengths of the client support systems.

Denial of impending loss or death is not a necessary condition of endings, and services that are cognizant of impending losses on a micro system level may facilitate the ending processes. Social workers should recognize physiological changes with approaching death (circulation, metabolism, secretions, respirations, elimination, and senses) and experiences with grief (mood, physical symptoms, sleep, appetite, energy, sensing a presence, preoccupations, or a need to care for someone). Attention to wills, funeral plans, and other personal business allows a greater focus on other choices in dying that are part of the endings process.

Workers need to be attuned to their own experiences with loss, endings, and grief. Workers may have feelings of guilt or remorse for the nonresponsive PWA to the promise of the medical "magical" cures. Workers may experience anger, blame, or frustration with the PWA for not making all the life choices. Avoidance and emotional distancing become defenses that carry workers through the pain of loss but tend to separate them from their work and the ones they help. Helping by instilling hope is a vital intervention technique, but extinguishable when the burden of loss is great. Care providers who cope best with loss are those who benefit the most from the experiences of caring. It becomes an organizational and community responsibility to help client systems deal with loss issues, including protecting workers (Davidson and Foster, 1995).

Values and Ethics

A host of ethical issues challenges the values of the profession in work with HIV/AIDS services. The core principles of ethical practice include justice, autonomy, beneficence, nonmaleficence, and fidelity (Beauchamp and Childress, 1989). In HIV care, these principles become challenged regarding issues of duty to treat; duty to warn; end of life issues; dual relationships; scarcity of resources; and confidentiality (Center for Substance Abuse Treatment, 2000). We need to know how we support the empowerment process in our work by recognizing ways ethical principles and professional values affect interactions with clients. Some issues are challenging, such as intentionally helping a suffering person to hasten death. Other value issues are more routine, such as protection of confidentiality. Ethical guidelines and foundations may help illuminate practice applications (Reamer, 1991a) as do policies and laws protecting medical confidentiality. When values clash, such as in confidentiality and the duty to warn (Reamer, 1991b), legal precedents and professional standards may be a guide as well as a liability protection. Sometimes workers are caught between the duty to maintain confidentiality yet work with the person to lessen potential risk to others. Workers may feel obligated to break confidentiality when a client gives them information about possible harm to others, such as engaging in at-risk sexual or drug-sharing behaviors. Workers often become involved in conflicting opinions, laws, and agency procedures about when and how to address duty to warn when it is in conflict with confidentiality standards. The conflict may appear to be between given interpretations of health codes, statutory regulations, case law, agency policy, and professional codes of conduct.

Unfortunately, much of the discussion about ethics in professional practice emphasizes micro (or individual level interactions) rather than macro system interactions. For example, relational boundary issues often arise because complaints are lodged at that level, and review panels are often dominated by micro-level practitioners. This holds practitioners accountable to individual complaints on a micro-level case basis, thus trivializing broader concerns with equity and distribution. Treatments can be costly, but they are effective; prevention is also cost effective (Creese et al., 2002). We need to examine such issues in the context of public good, and not consider just cost or effectiveness (Piot, Zewdie, and Tumen, 2002).

Complaints about relational boundary issues dominate ethical discussion, whereas discussions about cost/benefits or distributional justice in services are less likely to be addressed in professional literature. This limits the discussion of ethics and marginalizes those whose lives are endangered by health disparity outcomes. This context is also examined in a discussion of the care for persons with severe mental illness (Morse, Johnson, and Heyliger, 2000). It has implications for the discussion of ethical practice in HIV care as well.

The discussion of morality and ethics in practice unfortunately stays focused on micro system levels. This discussion would be better served by including multiple system levels and interactions, such as culture, gender, and larger issues of the responsibility of helping

(Abramson, 1996). The news media seem to obsess over sexual ethics on the individual level, and fail to articulate ethical concerns at a macro level, where many people are dying from AIDS daily. We have the capacity to respond with treatments, yet this is not at the core of the policy debate. Without a distributive social justice theme, limiting the discussions to micro-level ethics becomes sterile and disempowering. Unfortunately, health disparities are not as great an ethical concern as individual behavioral concerns. Such concerns limit the value of ethical practice discussions.

CONCLUSION

The empowerment of people is the most effective public health measure available. It is no longer possible, especially after the work of Jonathan Mann with the World Health Organization, to view medical care as separate from the struggle for human rights in such areas as women's equality, confidentiality, compulsory testing, and non-discrimination policies (Mann, 1992). Ethics regarding micro-level care delivery to individuals is an incomplete analysis without the links to distributive public health ethics on the macro level (Mann, 1997).

The miracles of HIV care are near—they are appearing in many cases in the United States. Hopes abound for new and better HIV treatments and vaccines, as well as new and civil rights laws to protect those affected. Overberg (1994) states that there remains but one answer to AIDS—compassion. Compassion for human rights becomes the tool for the delivery of public health services. Unless methods of prevention, with or without a vaccine, are successful, Fauci (2000) argues that the worst of the global pandemic will occur in the twenty-first century. Social work has a contribution to make, and it is made daily in generalist practice in which compassion and human rights produce better health and a better quality of life for people.

Considerable progress in HIV care and service delivery has been outlined in this chapter. Although no magic bullet for prevention has been developed, considerable progress has been made in prevention, treatments, and service delivery, which have expanded to reach a wide and growing population in need. The successes offer potential to improve the quality of life for those living with HIV. Having no cure has made life difficult for persons living with HIV and their loved ones, and it has made care delivery just as hard. Problems of access and of behavioral risk continue to elude effective prevention and adequate care. Progress on some fronts in treatments and psychosocial changes seems to reflect the miracles of success, as well as the shame of disparity and ineffectualness. Those who benefit from treatments live in the shadows of success, and those who do not benefit continue to die early and fast. Aronstein and Thompson (1998) discuss important concepts learned from this pandemic: live life more fully, do not make assumptions, listen to our clients, learn about courage from our clients, learn by our own limitations, and learn to take care of ourselves. In grappling with these lessons we learn how effectively our models of practice serve.

REFERENCES

Abramson, M. (1996). Toward a more holistic understanding of ethics in social work. *Social Work in Health Care, 23*(2), 1-14.

American Psychiatric Association (2000). *Practice guidelines for the treatment of patients with HIV/AIDS*. Washington, DC: American Psychiatric Association Press.

Andersen, R. M., Bozzette, S., Shapiro, M., St. Clair, P., Morton, S., Crystal, S., Goldman, D., Wenger, N., Gifford, A., and Leibowitz, A. (2000). Access of vulnerable groups to antiretroviral therapy among persons in care for HIV disease in the United States. *Health Services Research, 35*(2), 389-416.

Aronstein, D. M. and Thompson, B. J. (Eds.) (1998). *HIV and social work: A practitioners guide*. Binghamton, NY: The Haworth Press.

Bamberger, J. D., Unick, J., Klein, P., Fraser, M., Chesney, M., and Katz, M. H. (2000). Helping the urban poor stay with antiretroviral HIV drug therapy. *American Journal of Public Health, 90*(5), 699-701.

Bartlett, J. A. (2000). *Adherence and successful HIV management*. Chapel Hill, NC: Duke University School of Medicine, Office of Continuing Medical Education.

Bartlett, J. G. (2001). *Medical management of HIV infection*. Baltimore: Johns Hopkins University Press.

Battle, J. and Bennett, M. (2000). Research on lesbian and gay populations within the African American community: What have we learned? *African American Research Perspectives, 6*(2), 35-47.

Baumann, S. L. (1993). Mental health assessment of persons with HIV. *Nurses in AIDS Care, 4*(4), 36.

Beauchamp, T. L. and Childress, J. F. (1989). *Principles of biomedical ethics*, Third edition. New York: Oxford University Press.

Biestek, F. (1957). *The casework relationship.* Chicago, IL: Loyola University Press.

Binson, D. and Catania, J. A. (1998). Respondents' understanding of the words used in sexual behavior questions. *Public Opinion Quarterly, 62*(2), 190.

Blumberg, E. J., Hovell, M. F., Werner, C. A., Kelley, N. J., Sipan, C. L, Burkham, S. M., and Hofstetter, C. R. (1997). Evaluating AIDS-related social skills in Anglo and Latino adolescents. *Behavior Modification, 21*(3), 281-307.

Bonuck, K. A. (1993). AIDS and families: Cultural, psychosocial, and functional impacts. *Social Work in Health Care, 18*(2), 75-89.

Bor, R. and Miller, R. (1988). *AIDS: A guide to clinical counseling.* London: Science Press.

Briggs, L. P., Patnaude, P., Scavron, J., Whelan, M., and Etkind, P. (1995). The importance of social histories for assessing sexually transmitted disease risk. *Sexually Transmitted Disease, 22*(6), 348-350.

Brown, D. L. (1996). Living and working with HIV/AIDS: An empowerment model for community-based AIDS organizations and PWAs. Paper presented at the International AIDS Conference, July 7-12. Johnson City, New York: Southern Tier AIDS Programs, Inc.

Butters, N., Grant, I., Haxby, J., Judd, L. L., Martin, A., McClelland, J., Pequegnat, W., Schacter, D., and Stover, E. (1990). Assessment of AIDS-related cognitive changes: Recommendations of the NIMH workshop on neuropsychological assessment approaches. *Journal of Clinical and Experimental Neuropsychology, 12*(6), 963-978.

Bynum, R. (1998). Study finds infection rates higher for poor females age 16-21 than males. *Buffalo News,* August 28, p. 16A.

Cadman, J. (1998). Working to improve pregnancy outcomes. *Treatment Issues, 12*(7/8), 25-31.

Catania, J. A., Osmond, D., Stall, R. D., Pollack, L., Paul, J. P., Blower, S., Binson, D., Canchola, J. A., Mills, T. C., Fisher, L., et al. (2001). The continuing HIV epidemic among men who have sex with men. *American Journal of Public Health, 91*(6), 907-914.

CDC: Gay, bisexual men driving epidemic. (1999). *Washington Blade,* September 9, p. 1.

Center for Substance Abuse Treatment (CSAT) (2000). *Substance abuse treatment for persons living with HIV/AIDS.* Washington, DC: DHHS Publication (SMA 00-3410). This publication is one of the CSAT Treatment Improvement Protocol Series (#37).

Centers for Disease Control and Prevention (1999). *Compendium of HIV prevention interventions with evidence of effectiveness.* Atlanta, GA: Authors.

Centers for Disease Control and Prevention (2001). *HIV/AIDS Surveillance Report 13.* Atlanta, GA: Authors.

Chidwick, A. and Borrill, J. (1996). Dealing with life-threatening diagnosis: The experience of PWAs. *AIDS Care, 8*(3), 271-284.

Chuang, H. T., Devins, G. M., Hunsley, J., and Gill, M. J. (1989). Psychosocial distress and well-being among gay and bisexual men with HIV infection. *American Journal of Psychiatry, 146*(7), 876-880.

Clements-Nolle, K., Marx, R., Guzman, R., and Katz, M. (2001). HIV prevalence, risk behaviors, health care use, and mental health status of transgendered persons. *American Journal of Public Health, 91*(6), 915-921.

Clifford, R. (1997). Managing mental health care. *Focus, 12*(12), 5-6.

Cohen, D., Scribner, R., Redimo, R., and Farley, T. A. (2000). Domestic violence and childhood sexual abuse in HIV infected women and women at risk for HIV. *American Journal of Public Health, 90*(4), 560-567.

Cohen, J. (2001). *Shots in the dark: The wayward search for an AIDS vaccine.* New York: W. W. Norton Company.

Cohler, B. J. and Galatzer-Levy, R. M. (2000). *The course of gay and lesbian lives: Social and psychoanalytic perspectives.* Chicago: University of Chicago Press.

Collins, E., Wagner, C., and Walmsley, S. (2000). Psychosocial impact of the lipodystrophy syndrome in HIV infection. *The AIDS Reader, 10*(9), 546-551.

Creese, A., Floyd, K., Alban, A., and Guinness, L. (2002). Cost-effectiveness of HIV/AIDS interventions in Africa: A systematic review of the evidence. *Lancet, 359,* 1635-1642.

Cunningham, W. E. (2002). Participation in research and access to experimental treatments for HIV-infected patients. *NEJM, 346*(18), 1373-1382.

Davidson, K. W. and Foster, Z. (1995). Social work with dying and bereaved clients: Helping the workers. *Health and Social Work, 21*(4), 1-16.

Dean, H. D., Fleming, P. L., and Ward, J. W. (1993). Recent trends among Black and Hispanic adults with AIDS in the United States: 1988-1991. Atlanta, GA: Centers for Disease Control and Prevention, published in AIDSLine.

Diaz, T., Buehler, J. W., Castro, K. G., and Ward, J. W. (1993). AIDS trends among Hispanics in the United States. *American Journal of Public Health, 83*(4), 504-509.

Dicks, B. A. (1994). African-American women and AIDS: A public health/social work challenge. *Social Work in Health Care, 19*(3/4), 123-143.

Dilley, J. W., Pies, C., and Helquist, M. (1993). *Face to face: A guide to AIDS counseling.* San Francisco, CA: UCSF AIDS Health Plan.

DiPasquale, J. A. (1990). The psychological effects of support groups on individuals infected by the AIDS virus. *Cancer Nursing, 13*(5), 278-285.

Edwards, E., Shachter, A., and Owens, D. K. (1998). A dynamic HIV transmission model for evaluating the costs and benefits of vaccine programs. *Interfaces, 28*(3), 144.

Fauci, A. S. (2000). The AIDS epidemic: Considerations for the 21st century. *Global Issues: An Electronic Journal of the U. S. Department of State, 5*(2), 1-12.

Fox, K. K., del Rio, C., Holmes, K. K., Hook, E. W., Judson, F. N., Knapp, J. S., Procop, G. W., Wang, S. A., Whittington, W. L., and Levine, W. C. (2001). Gonorrhea in the HIV era: A reversal in trends among men who have sex with men. *American Journal of Public Health, 91*(6), 959-964.

Friedmann, P. D., McCullough, M. S., and Saitz, R. (2001). Screening and intervention for illicit drug abuse. *Archives of Internal Medicine, 161*, 248-251.

Garnet, L. D. and D'Augelli, A. R. (1994). Empowering lesbian and gay communities: A call for collaboration with community psychology. *American Journal of Community Psychology, 22*(4), 447-470.

Garrett, L. (1994). *The coming plague: Newly emerging diseases in a world out of balance.* New York: Penguin Books.

Gates, H. L. (1998). Backlash? All prejudices are not equal. But that doesn't mean there's no comparison between the predicaments of gays and blacks. *The New Yorker Magazine,* May 17.

Germain, C. B. and Gitterman, A. (1995). *The life model of social work practice,* Second edition. New York: Columbia University Press.

Gilden, D., Falkenberg, J., and Torres, G. (1997). Protease inhibitors: Resistance, resistance, resistance. *Treatment Issues, 11*(2), 1-6.

Goicoechea-Balbona, A. M. (1997). Culturally specific health care model for ensuring health care use by rural, ethnically diverse families affected by AIDS. *Health and Social Work, 22*(3), 172-180.

Goicoechea-Balbona, A. M. (1998). Children with HIV/AIDS and their families: A successful social work intervention based on the culturally specific health care model. *Health and Social Work, 23*(1), 61-69.

Goodman, R. M., Wandersman, A., Chinman, M., Imm, P., and Morrissey, E. (1996). An ecological assessment of community-based interventions for prevention and health promotion. *American Journal of Community Psychology, 24*(1), 33-61.

Gore-Felton, C. and Spiegel, D. (1999). Enhancing women's lives: The role of support groups among breast cancer patients. *Journal of Specialists in Group Work, 24*(3), 274-287.

Greenstein, M. and Breitbart, W. (2000). Cancer and experience of meaning: A group psychotherapy program for people with cancer. *American Journal of Psychotherapy, 54*(4), 486-500.

Gutheil, I. A. and Chichin, E. R. (1991). AIDS, older people, and social work. *Health and Social Work, 16*(4), 237-144.

Gutierrez, L. (1989). Empowerment in social work practice. Paper presented at the Council on Social Work Education, Annual Program, Chicago, Illinois.

Haney, D. Q. (1998). AIDS treatment fails many patients. Baltimore, MD: Associated Press Report, August 22.

Hanson, G. R. (2002). NIDA research advances global efforts to prevent and treat AIDS. *NIDA Notes, 17*(1), 3-4.

Hartman, A. and Laird, J. (1983). *Family-centered social work practice.* New York: Free Press.

Hecht, F. M. (1998). Measuring HIV treatment adherence in clinical practice. *AIDS Clinical Care, 10*(8), 1.

Heckman, T. (2000). Older patients with HIV depressed, suicidal. *Psychiatric Services,* June 27, 5.

Heimer, R. (1998). Syringe exchange programs. *Public Health, 113,* supplement, 67.

HIV incidence among young men who have sex with men—Seven United States cities, 1994-2000. (2001). *MMWR, 50,* 440-444.

HIV prevention through case management for HIV-infected persons—selected sites, United States, 1989-1992. (1993). *MMWR, 44,* 448.

HIV/AIDS Bureau (2000). *The AIDS epidemic and the Ryan White Care Act.* Washington, DC: USFHHS Publication. Article can also be found online at: <http://hab.hrsa.gov/ryan/index.html>.

Hoffman, K. S. and Sallee, A. L. (1993). *Social work practice: Bridges to change.* Boston: Allyn & Bacon Press.

Holmes, K. A. and Hodge, R. H. (1995). Gay and lesbian persons. In J. Philleo and F. L. Brisbane (Eds.), *Cultural competence for social workers* (pp. 191-218). Washington, DC: Centers for Substance Abuse Prevention.

Hooper, L. (2000). 80 percent of HIV patients in study take medication improperly. *Houston Chronicle,* July 14, p. 22A.

Icard, L. K., Schilling, R. F., el-Bassel, N., and Young, D. (1992). Preventing AIDS among black gay men and black gay and heterosexual male intravenous drug users. *Social Work, 37*(5), 440-445.

Ickovics, J. (2001). Depression linked to HIV progression. *Journal of the American Medical Association, 285,* 1466-1474.

Indyk, D., Belville, R., Lachapelle, S., Gordon, G., and Dewart, T. (1993). A community-based approach to HIV case management: Systematizing the unmanageable. *Social Work, 38*(4), 380-387.

James, J. S. (2000). Many people with HIV/AIDS not getting proper treatment. *AIDS Treatment News, 354*(3), 1.

Johnson, L. C. (1988). *Social work practice: A generalist perspective,* Sixth edition. Boston: Allyn & Bacon Press.

Joslin, D. and Brouard, A. (1995). The prevalence of grandmothers as primary care givers in a poor pediatric population. *Journal of Community Health, 20*(5), 383-401.

Kaiser Family Foundation. (2002). *The global impact of HIV/AIDS in youth: An HIV/AIDS policy fact sheet.* Available online at: <http://www.kff.org>.

Karon, J. M., Fleming, P. L., Steketee, R. W., and de Cock, K. M. (2001). HIV in the US at the turn of the century. *Americal Journal of Public Health, 91*(7), 1060-1068.

Katz, M. H., Cunningham, W. E., Fleishman, J. A., Andersen, R. M., Kellog, T., Bozzette, S. A., and Shapiro, M. A. (2001). Effects of case management on unmet needs and utilization of medical care and medications among HIV-infected persons. *Annals of Internal Medicine, 135,* October 16, 610-612.

Katz, M. H., Douglas, J. M., Bolan, G. A., Marx, R., Sweat, S. M., Park, M. S., and Buchbinder, S. P. (1996). Depression and use of mental health services among HIV-infected men. *AIDS Care, 8*(4), 433-442.

Kelly, J. A., Somlai, A. M., DiFranciesco, W. J., Oho-Salaj, L. L., McAuliffe, T. L., Hackl, K. L., Heckman, T. G., Holtgrave, P. R., and Rompa, D. (2000). Bridging the gap between the science and service of HIV prevention: Transferring effective research-based HIV prevention interventions to community AIDS service providers. *American Journal of Public Health, 90*(7), 1082-1088.

Kendall, J. (1996). Human association as a factor influencing wellness in homosexual men with HIV disease. *Applied Nursing Research, 9*(4), 195-203.

Klein, S. J., Birkhead, G. S., and Wright, G. (2000). Domestic violence and HIV/AIDS (Letter to the Editor). *American Journal of Public Health, 90*, 1648.

Koetting, M. E. (1996). A group design for HIV-negative gay men. *Social Work, 41*(4), 407-415.

Kolata, G. (2002). Research suggests more health care may not be better. *The New York Times,* July 21, p. 1.

Lee, L. M., Karon, J. M., and Selik, R. (2001). Survival after AIDS diagnosis in adolescents and adults during the treatment era, United States, 1984-1997. *Journal of the American Medical Association, 285*(10), 1308.

Leserman, J. (1999). Lack of social support may cause HIV+ men to develop AIDS more quickly. *Psychosomatic Medicine, 61*(3), 397-406.

Leserman, J. (2000). Denial and stress speed progression of HIV to AIDS. *American Journal of Psychiatry, 157*, 1221-1228.

Levin, A. (1998). 97 AIDS claims under $1 billion. *National Underwriter, 102*(34), 1.

Levin, S. (1998). Triple therapy leads to HIV treatment options. *HealthWire.* January 27.

Link, D. (1999). Medicaid managed care and people with HIV. *GMHC Treatment Issues, 13*(7/8), 5.

Lippmann, S. B., James, W. A., and Frierson, R. L. (1993). AIDS and the family: Implications for counseling. *AIDS Care, 5*(1), 71-78.

Lishner, D. M., Richardson, M., Levine, P., and Patrick, D. (1996). Access to primary health care among persons with disabilities in rural areas: A summary of the literature. *Journal of Rural Health, 12*(1), 45-53.

Louisiana Office of Public Health (1998). Adult AIDS cases by gender, ethnicity and exposure category. *HIV/AIDS Line 7*(4), 5.

Lutgendorf, S., Antoni, M. H., Schneiderman, N., and Fletcher, M. A. (1994). Psychosocial counseling to improve the quality of life in HIV infection. *Patient Education and Counseling, 24*(3), 217-235.

Lynch, V. J., Lloyd, G. A., and Fimbres, M. F. (1993). *The changing face of AIDS: Implications for social work practice.* Westport, CT: Auburn House.

Magen, R. H. and Glajchen, M. (1999). Cancer support groups: Client outcomes and context of group process. *Research on Social Work Practice, 9*(5), 541-554.

Mancoske, R. J. (1997a). The international AIDS crisis. In M. C. Hokenstad and J. Midgley (Eds.), *Issues in international social work* (pp. 125-145). Washington, DC: National Association of Social Workers Press.

Mancoske, R. J. (1997b). Rural HIV/AIDS social services for gays and lesbians. In J. D. Smith and R. J. Mancoske (Eds.), *Rural gays and lesbians: Building on community strengths* (pp. 37-52). Binghamton, NY: The Haworth Press.

Mancoske, R. J. and Hunzeker, J. M. (1990). *Empowerment based generalist practice: Direct services with individuals* (revised). New York: Cummings and Hathaway Press.

Mancoske, R. J. and Lindhorst, T. (1994). Group work practice in an HIV/AIDS outpatient clinic. In M. M. Campbell (Ed.), *Social group work in the 1990s* (Volume 19) (pp. 71-81). New Orleans, LA: Tulane University Studies in Social Welfare.

Mancoske, R. J. and Lindhorst, T. (1995). The ecological context of HIV/AIDS counseling. In G. A. Lloyd and M. A. Kuszelewicz (Eds.), *HIV disease: Lesbians, gays, and social services* (pp. 41-60). Binghamton, NY: The Haworth Press.

Mancoske, R. J., Waddsworth, C. M., Dugas, D. S., and Hasney, J. A. (1995). Suicide risk among PWAs. *Social Work, 40*(6), 783-788.

Mann, J. M. (1992). AIDS and human rights. In J. M. Mann, D. J. M. Tatantolla, and T. W. Netter (Eds.), *AIDS in the world* (pp. 537-574). Cambridge, MA: Harvard University Press.

Mann, J. M. (1997). Medicine, and public health, ethics and human rights. *Hastings Center Report, 27*(3), 6-13.

Maris, R. W., Berman, A. L., Maltsberger, J. T., and Yufit, R. I. (1992). *Assessment and prediction of suicide.* New York: Guilford Press.

Markowitz, J. C., Kocsis, J. H., Fishman, B., Spielman, L. A., Jacobsberg, L. B., Frances, A. J., Klerrman, G. L., and Perry, S. W. (1998). Treatment of depressive symptoms in HIV-positive patients. *Archives of General Psychiatry, 55*(3), 452-457.

Marx, R., Katz, M. H., Park, M. S., and Gurley, R. J. (1997). Meeting the service needs of HIV-infected persons: Is Ryan White Care Act succeeding? *Journal of AIDS and Human Retro- viruses, 14*(1), 44-55.

McCaffrey, B. R. (1998). Drug treatment: Cost effective and humane. *Washington Post,* September 1, A-18.

McDonell, J. R., Abell, N., and Miller, J. (1991). Family members' willingness to care for people with AIDS: A psychosocial assessment model. *Social Work, 36*(1), 43-53.

McGlynn, E. A. and Brook, R. H. (1996). Ensuring quality of care. In R. M. Andersen, T. H. Rice, and G. F. Kominski (Eds.), *Changing the U.S. health care system* (pp. 142-179). San Francisco, CA: Jossey-Bass.

McKeown, L. A. (2001). U.S. women increasingly infected by HIV: African Americans living in Southern states have highest infection rates. This article is discussing an article in a March 7, 2001 article in the *Journal of the American*

Medical Association by S. Hader and found at the WebMD Medical News online at: <http://ww2.aegis.org/news/webmd/2001/WM010301.html>.

McMahon, M. O. (1995). *The general method of social work practice: A generalist perspective.* Upper Saddle River, NJ: Pearson, Allyn, and Bacon.

McMillan, C. (1988). Families in crisis: Coping with AIDS. *Focus, 3*(10), 1.

Mellins, C. A. and Ehrhardt, A. A. (1994). Families affected by pediatric AIDS: Sources of stress and coping. *Journal of Developmental Behavioral Pediatrics, 15*(3), 54-60.

Metzger, D. S., Navaline, H., and Woody, G. E. (1998). Drug abuse treatment and AIDS preventions. *Public Health, 113,* (supplement) 1.

Meyer, C. H. and Mattaini, M. A. (Eds.) (1995). *The foundations of social work practice.* Silver Spring, MD: National Association of Social Workers Press.

Miley, K. K., O'Melia, M., and Dubois, B. (1998). *Generalist social work practice: An empowering approach,* Second edition. Boston: Allyn & Bacon Press.

Montgomery, J. P., Gillespie, B. W., Gentry, A. C., Mokotoff, E. D., Crane, L. R., and James, S. A. (2002). Does access to health care impact survival time after diagnosis of AIDS? *AIDS Patient Care and STDs, 16*(5), 223-231.

Morrison, C. S., McCusker, J., Stoddard, A. M., and Bigelow, C. (1995). The validity of behavioral data reported by injection drug users on a clinical risk assessment. *International Journal of Addictions, 30*(7), 889-899.

Morse, J. K., Johnson, D. J., and Heyliger, S. O. (2000). Understanding ethnic disparities in the treatment of affective disorders. *Minority Health Today, 2*(1), 24-27.

Motto, J. A. (1991). An integrated approach to estimating suicide risk. *Suicide and Life Threatening Behavior, 21*(1), 74-89.

Nathanson, N. (1998). Harnessing research to control AIDS. *Nature Medicine, 4*(8), 879.

National Abandoned Infants Resource Center (2002). Mental health challenges among women, adolescents, and children living with HIV. *The Source, 11*(2), 1-4, 30.

National Institute on Drug Abuse (NIDA) (2000). *The NIDA community-based outreach model: A manual to reduce the risk of HIV and other blood-borne infections in drug users.* Washington, DC: National Clearinghouse for Alcohol and Drug Information.

National Institute on Drug Abuse (NIDA) (2002). *Principles of HIV prevention in drug-using populations: A research-based guide.* Washington, DC: Authors.

National Institute of Mental Health (NIMH) (2002). Depression and HIV/AIDS. Available online at: <www.nimh.gov/publicat/dephiv.cfm>.

Needle, R. H., Coyle, S. L., and Normand, J. (1998). HIV prevention with drug-using populations—Current status and future prospects: Introduction and overview. *Public Health, 113,* (supplement) 1-87.

No AIDS obits is news for gay paper, (1998). *Washington Post,* August 16, p. A7.

Northen, H. (1994). *Clinical social work knowledge and skills,* Second edition. New York: Columbia University Press.

Office of Minority Health (2001). HIV in prisons. *HIV impact.* Washington, DC: OMH, USDHHS, Authors.

Orgnero, M. K. and Rodway, M. R. (1991). AIDS and a social work treatment: A single-system design. *Health and Social Work, 16*(2), 123-141.

Overberg, K. R. (1994). *AIDS, ethics and religion: Embracing a world of suffering.* Maryknoll, NY: Orbis Books.

Owens, D. K., Brandeau, M. L., and Sox, C. H. (1996). Effect of relapse to high-risk behavior on the costs and benefits of a program to screen women for HIV. *Interfaces, 28*(3), 52.

Page, B. J., Delmonico, D. L., Walsh, J., and Amoreaux, N. A. (2000). Setting up online support groups using the Palace software. *Journal for Specialists in Group Work, 25*(2), 133-145.

Paterson, D. L., Swindells, S., Mohr, J., Brester, M., Vergis, E. N., Squier, C., Wagener, M., and Singh, N. (2000). Adherence to protease inhibitor therapy and outcomes in patients with HIV infection. *Annals of Internal Medicine, 133,* 21-30.

Pawlusiak, C. and Hickman, L. (1996). Community based HIV/AIDS case management services and corresponding cost reductions in inpatient hospitalization. Paper presented at the International Conference on AIDS, Harper Hospital, Detroit, Michigan, July 7-12.

Perlman, H. H. (1979). *Relationship: The heart of helping people.* Chicago, IL: University of Chicago Press.

Piot, P., Zewdie, D., and Tumen, T. (2002). HIV/AIDS prevention and treatment. *Lancet, 360,* 86-89.

Pizzi, M. (1992). Women, HIV infection, and AIDS: Tapestries of life, death and empowerment. *American Journal of Occupational Therapy, 46*(11), 1021-1027.

Presidential Advisory Council on HIV/AIDS (2000). *AIDS: No time to spare.* Washington, DC: Office of the White House.

The public health challenges of the HIV epidemic (2000). *American Journal of Public Health, 90*(7), 1023-1024.

Purdy, B. D. (2000). Medication errors in the HIV-infected population. *Medscape Pharmacist, 1*(6), 7403. Available online at: <http://www.medscape.com>.

Rayner-Brosnan, D. (1995). Wellness and HIV. *International Journal of Immunopharmacology, 17*(8), 663-676.

Reamer, F. (1991a). *AIDS and ethics.* New York: Columbia University Press.

Reamer, F. (1991b). AIDS and the duty to protect. *Social Work, 36*(1), 56-60.

Remafedi, G., French, S., Story, M., Resnick, M. D., and Blum, R. (1998). The relationship between suicide risk and sexual orientation: Results of a population based study. *American Journal of Public Health, 88*(1), 57-60.

Roberts, C. S., Severinson, C., Kuehn, C., Straker, D., Fritz, C. J., and Moffitt, H. L. (1992). Obstacles to effective case management with AIDS patients. *Social Work in Health Care, 17*(2), 27-40.

Rolland, J. S. (1994). *Families, illness, and disability: An integrative treatment model.* New York: Basic Books.

Rosenberg, S. D. Goodman, L. A., Osher, F. C., Swartz, M. S., Essock, S. M., Butterfield, M. I., Constantine, N. T., Wolford, G. L., and Salyers, M. P. (2001). Prevalence of HIV, HBC, HCV in people with severe mental illness. *American Journal of Public Health, 91*(1), 31-37.

Roth, J., Siegel, R., and Black, S. (1994). Identifying the mental health needs of children living in families with AIDS or HIV infection. *Community Mental Health Journal, 30*(6), 581-593.

Rothman, J. and Sager, J. S. (1998). *Case management: Integrating individual and community practice,* Second edition. Boston: Allyn & Bacon Press.

Samarel, N., Fawcett, J., and Tulman, L. (1997). Effect of support groups with coaching on adaptation to early stage breast cancer. *Research in Nursing and Health, 20*(1), 15-26.

Shapiro, M. F., Morton, S. C., McCaffrey, D. F., Senterfitt, J. W., Fleishman, J. A., Perlman, J. F., Athey, L. A., Keesey, J. W., Goldman, D. P., Berry, S. H., et al. (1999). Variations in the core of HIV infected adults in the United States: Results from the HIV cost and service utilization study. *Journal of the American Medical Association, 281*(24), 2305-2315.

Shelton, D. L. (2000). Complications of AIDS. *American Medical News, 43*(35), 25.

Shernoff, M. (1998). Getting started: Basic skills for effective social work with persons living with HIV/AIDS. In D. M. Aronson and B. J. Thompson (Eds.), *HIV and social work* (pp. 27-50). Binghamton, NY: The Haworth Press.

Shilts, R. (1987). *And the band played on: Politics, people and the AIDS epidemic.* New York: St. Martin's Press.

Sholevar, G. P. and Perkel, R. (1990). Family systems intervention and physical illness. *General Hospital Psychiatry, 12*(6), 363-372.

Singh, N., Squier, C., Sivek, C., Wagener, M., Nguyen, M. H., and Yu, V. L. (1996). Determinants of compliance with antiretroviral therapy in patients with HIV. *AIDS Care, 8*(3), 261-269.

Smith, J. D. and Mancoske, R. J. (1997). *Rural gays and lesbians: Building on community strengths.* Binghamton, NY: The Haworth Press.

Snell, C. L. (1995). *Young men in the street: Help seeking behavior of young male prostitutes.* Westport, CT: Praeger Press.

Solomon, B. (1976). *Black empowerment: Social work in oppressed communities.* New York: Columbia University Press.

Sontag, S. (1988). *AIDS as metaphor.* New York: Farrar, Giroux and Strauss Publishers.

Sorensen, J. L. and Miller, M. S. (1996). Impact of HIV risk and infection on delivery of psychosocial treatment services in outpatient programs. *Journal of Substance Abuse Treatment, 13*(5), 387-395.

Sowell, R. L. and Meadows, T. M. (1994). An integrated case management model: Developing standards, evaluation, and outcome criteria. *Nursing Administration, 18*(2), 53-64.

Spiegel, D., Kraemer, H. C., Bloom, J. R., and Gutheil, E. (1989). Effect of psychosocial treatment on survival of patients with metastatic breast cancer. *The Lancet, 355,* 888-891.

Spirig, R. (1998). Support groups for people living with HIV/AIDS: A review of the literature. *Journal of the Association of Nurses in AIDS Care, 9*(4), 44-57.

Stein, M. D. Crystal, S., Cunningham, W. E., Ananthanarayanan, A., Andersen, R. M., Turner, B. J., Zierler, S., Morton, S., Katz, M. H., Bozzette, S., et al. (2000). Delays in seeking HIV care due to competing care giver responsibilities. *American Journal of Public Health, 90*(7), 1138-1144.

Stephensen, J. (2002). Sobering levels of drug resistent HIV found. *JAMA, 287*(6), 1021.

Sternberg, S. (1998). Teenagers in turmoil. *USA Today,* October 5, p. D1.

Sternberg, S. (2001). "Secret" bisexuality among Black men contributing to rising number of AIDS cases in Black women. *USA Today,* March 15, p. D1.

Substance Abuse and Mental Health Services Administration (1998). *Services research outcomes study.* Washington, DC: Authors.

Taylor-Brown, S. and Garcia, A. (1995). Social workers and HIV-affected families: Is the profession prepared? *Social Work, 40*(1), 14-15.

Teenagers at risk (1998). *Washington Post,* August 25, p. A5.

Texeira, E. (1998). US adds $4.9 million to funds aimed at AIDS and minorities. *Baltimore Sun,* September 8, A3.

Tolson, J. (2000). Access to triple HIV therapy might reduce cost of treating opportunistic infections. *Journal of AIDS, 26,* 302-313.

Topping, S., Hartwig, L. C., and Cecil, A. (1997). Delivering care to rural HIV/AIDS patients. *Journal of Rural Health, 13*(3), 226-236.

Undeterred by a monster: Secrecy and stigma keep AIDS high risk for gay black men (2001). *The New York Times,* February 11, p. 37.

United Nations Economic and Social Council (2002). *Report on the global impact of the HIV/AIDS epidemic.* New York: Authors.

United Nations Global AIDS Program (2002). UN Fact Sheet. Available online at: <www.unaids.org/fact_sheets/files>.

Valentich, M. (1986). Feminism and social work practiced. In F. Turner (Ed.), *Social work treatment,* Third edition (pp. 564-589). New York: Free Press.

Viorst, J. (1986). *Necessary losses.* New York: Ballantine Books.

Walkup, J., Crystal, S., and Sambamoorthi, U. (1999). Schizophrenia and major affective disorders among Medicaid recipients with HIV/AIDS in New Jersey. *American Journal of Public Health, 89*(7), 1101-1103.

Weinhardt, L. S., Carey, M. P., Johnson, B. T., and Bickham, N. L. (1999). Effects of HIV counseling and testing on sexual risk behavior: A meta-analysis review of published research, 1985-1997. *American Journal of Public Health, 89*(9), 1397-1405.

White House Report (2000). *Youth and HIV/AIDS 2000: A new American agenda.* Washington, DC: Authors.

Williams, D. R. and Rucker, T. D. (2000). Understanding and addressing racial disparities in health care. *Minority Health Today, 2*(1), 30-39.

Wilson, P. A. (1995). AIDS service organizations: Current issues and future challenges. In G. A. Lloyd and M. A. Kuszelewicz (Eds.), *HIV disease: Lesbians, gays and the social services* (pp. 121-144). Binghamton, NY: The Haworth Press.

Woodman, N. (1989). Mental health issues of relevance to lesbian women and gay men. *Journal of Lesbian and Gay Psychotherapy, 1*(1), 53-64.

Zaric, G. S., Barnett, P. G., and Brandeau, M. L. (2000). HIV transmission and cost-effectiveness of methadone maintenance. *American Journal of Public Health, 90*(7), 1100-1111.

Chapter 2

Case Management

DeAnn Gruber

INTRODUCTION

Shortly after HIV/AIDS reached epidemic proportions in vulnerable populations during the mid-1980s, it was quickly identified that a variety of medical and social services were needed to improve HIV-infected individuals' chances for longer life. Case management was accepted as a critical component of the continuum of care for persons living with HIV/AIDS. Throughout the country, AIDS service organizations implemented models of case management to increase access to needed services. However, a variety of models, standards of care, and evaluation strategies were adopted for this population. This chapter provides a summary of the varying models of case management and how these models may differ among populations, with an emphasis on the development and provision of case management for persons living with HIV/AIDS. Furthermore, it explores how research in this field has influenced the development and implementation of effective case management services. Thus, a review of the body of research conducted to determine the effectiveness of case management will be presented, how this impacts practitioners, in addition to a discussion of areas that need further exploration in this field.

CASE MANAGEMENT MODELS

History

During the past thirty years, the topic of case management has been thoroughly presented in the literature. According to Vourlekis

(1992), the interest in case management for certain populations is pervasive in all fields, cutting across the public and private sectors. Settings that utilize case management have expanded to include schools, health and mental health clinics, hospitals, businesses, and major insurance companies. During the 1970s, a number of major public programs using case management services were initiated. Medicare and Medicaid waivers authorized research and demonstration projects in the provision of community-based care for the frail elderly as an alternative to costly institutionalized care. Case management was also a required component of demonstration projects to facilitate client access to appropriate services in what had come to be acknowledged as a fragmented and bewildering health and social services delivery system (Austin et al.,1985). With the onset of deinstitutionalization of chronically mentally ill individuals, correlated with the increasing attention directed to the deficiencies of community mental health centers, case management was introduced as a component of service delivery. Similar programs followed for the developmentally disabled, homeless, and children with special needs.

Definition and Functions of Case Management

Although definitions of case management abound, Sowell and Grier (1995, p. 15) describe it as a "client-focused process that augments and coordinates existing services." One goal of case management is to optimize client functioning by providing quality services in the most efficient and effective manner to individuals with multiple complex needs (National Association of Social Workers, 1992); improving a client's quality of life is emphasized as an outcome of this goal. A second goal of case management is related to cost containment, with the anticipation that the provision of case management services will reduce the use of expensive inpatient care, allowing resources to be allocated in an efficient manner (Chernesky, 1999; Katz et al., 2000; Piette et al., 1995; Rothman, 1994).

Unfortunately, these two goals can work against each other, forcing case managers to choose between various roles, such as a broker, in which case resources must be managed and services are rationed to reduce costs. An alternative role is that of advocate, in which case managers identify gaps and advocate for improved services based on need (Moore, 1992; Raiff and Shore, 1993). In fact, Netting (1992) proposed that this tension is rooted in early social work history, when the Charity Organization Societies focused on guarding the dollars or assuming the gatekeeper role, whereas proponents of the settlement house movement focused on assisting poor individuals through an advocacy role.

In 1992, the National Association of Social Workers adopted a definition of *social work case management:* a method of providing services whereby a professional social worker assesses the needs of the client and the client's family, when appropriate, and arranges, coordinates, monitors, evaluates, and advocates for a package of multiple services to meet the specific client's complex needs (NASW, 1992). Distinct from other forms of case management, social work case management addresses both the individual client's biopsychosocial status, as well as the state of the social system in which case management operates.

The field has identified and adopted five basic functions of case management:

1. outreach to or identification of clients;
2. assessment;
3. service or treatment planning;
4. linking or referring clients to appropriate resources; and
5. monitoring of cases to ensure that services are delivered and used (Piette et al., 1995; Rose and Moore, 1995).

Additional functions in comprehensive case management models include resource identification, advocacy, evaluation, and termination (NASW, 1992; Raiff and Shore, 1993; Vourlekis, 1992; Weil and Karls, 1985). Rothman (1994) elaborates his model by including a total of fifteen different functions: in addition to those previously listed, he also proposes that counseling/therapy, reassessment, and interagency coordination are essential case management tasks.

Practice Models of Case Management

Varying models of case management have been developed during the past thirty years because of the range of agreement regarding the specific functions and activities of case managers. However, three primary practice models have emerged in the field. The broker model and the therapeutic or clinical model emphasize the particular goals and activities of case management, as well as the needed skill level of the staffperson providing these services. The third model, assertive community treatment, utilizes a team approach, primarily in the mental health field and will also be described, since it has been recognized as an effective practice model in the literature.

The classic broker model of case management focuses on activities that will increase clients' linkage to services, in order to improve their overall functioning and quality of life. Contacts with clients are typically brief, reactive, and allow minimal affective involvement between the client and case manager. Instead, when a medical and/or psychosocial need is identified, the case manager is contacted by the client and resources are arranged. Although follow-up and monitoring of the client's progress in accessing these services are expected, a case manager's role in maintaining contact over time is limited. Many times caseloads are large, which also reinforces the practice of not developing a therapeutic relationship with the client; subsequently, educational and skill level standards of case managers in a broker model are not high.

The therapeutic or clinical model of case management expands the role of the case manager from simple broker to treatment provider. In this approach, the relationship that is established between the case manager and client is a therapeutic intervention in itself, which aids in the helping process for the client. Thus, in addition to coordinating a client's care, identifying service needs, and linking the client to available resources, the rapport and trust that is established between the client and case manager is "a mode of therapy in itself" (Harris and Bergman, 1987, p. 296). Different from the broker model, this approach is proactive and de-emphasizes activities related to community development, advocacy, and outreach. Case managers are highly trained and caseloads are smaller to provide additional time for developing the therapeutic relationship.

A third case management approach is the therapeutic team approach or assertive community treatment (ACT). This model emerged during the 1970s, based on Stein and Test's work with Wisconsin's Program for Assertive Community Treatment (Stein and Test, 1980). The unique element in this approach is the utilization of multidisciplinary teams to provide a range of specialty services to clients, with the intent to reduce unnecessary hospitalizations and to improve the client's independent functioning in the community.

Pescosolido, Wright, and Sullivan (1995) identify four assumptions to the ACT case management approach. The first assumption is the notion that a multidisciplinary team of providers can conduct a more thorough assessment of needs with the client and identify issues that may be overlooked by others. Another assumption of the ACT approach is that inherent benefits may be reaped by staff as individual members of a team. For example, staff burnout may be prevented due to the shared responsibility and support that occurs within a team setting. The third assumption is that disruption may be minimized when a staffperson leaves; in the ACT model, since several individuals are involved in the client's treatment, the case management process may continue with the other team members. The final assumption is that again, since there is a shared accountability among team members, a client will be less likely to get lost in the system. Instead, increased instances of follow-up and contact will occur with the client, and hopefully, if a client begins to experience some potential social and psychological difficulty that impacts his or her functioning, prompt interventions by the case management team will occur.

Case Management Models for Persons Living with HIV/AIDS

In the arena of HIV/AIDS, the literature includes descriptive and evaluative studies regarding how case management services have been instrumental in increasing access to needed primary medical care and social support (Emlet and Guaz, 1998; Indyk et al., 1993; Katz et al., 2000; Littrell, 1998; Piette et al., 1995). Delivery of case management services to persons living with HIV/AIDS does not vary significantly from case management models for other populations. In fact, Piette and colleagues (1992) identified that HIV-infected individuals share common issues to two other groups that have traditionally benefited from case management: drug use, poverty, and discrimination are common issues for the chronically mentally ill, and waning physical capacity and the need for medical resources are prevailing problems for the elderly.

Due to limited resources and a delay from traditional social service organizations to adequately respond to the AIDS crisis in this country, volunteer-based agencies were established during the initial years of the epidemic. Thus, individuals with minimal social work experience were responsible for providing an array of services, including case management, to people with HIV. For example, in 1988, the Robert Wood Johnson Foundation funded ten demonstration projects in nine cities to develop comprehensive services for HIV-infected individuals. An evaluation study of these projects (Piette et al., 1992) reported that three sites implemented a community-based approach to case management service delivery. In these sites, services were frequently conducted by staff with little or no social work training. However, in the remaining projects, which were hospital- or clinic-based, many of the staff were health care professionals, including nurses and social workers.

Chernesky and Grube (2000) conducted a recent study to examine how HIV/AIDS case management services were implemented among fourteen AIDS service organizations. Utilizing the data collection methods of chart reviews and focus groups with case managers and program supervisors, Chernesky and Grube recognized eight themes related to case management. Clients receiving case management services were identified as highly vulnerable, meaning that HIV/AIDS was only one of multiple life stressors. For example, many individuals also faced inadequate housing, poverty, emotional isolation, and poor coping skills. The study also found that the case management process focused on two different components: crisis management and "maintenance management," a term coined by the study's authors. Case managers primarily concentrated on achieving a level of stability for clients during crises, rather than engaging in various noncrisis activities with clients. Many of these noncrisis tasks, including ongoing assessment and monitoring of clients' status and progress, service coordination, and continuous collaboration with providers are typically recognized as critical case management functions. Yet, in this study, case managers found that crisis management activities consumed the majority of their time, leaving little time available for other caseload maintenance activities.

Another theme supported by this and other studies (Austin, 1993; Moore, 1992; Netting, 1992; O'Connor, 1988), is the interaction of case management and the service delivery system or established provider network. Many times, the availability of resources, as well as the level of service coordination, will define the package of services that a case manager may provide to his or her clients. Thus, improving relationships among providers and advocating for increased resources are activities case managers perform, although they may not be universally identified as primary tasks or functions in the formal case management process.

RESEARCH OF CASE MANAGEMENT

During recent years, researchers have attempted to conduct studies to assess the effectiveness of case management services provided to varying populations. The following section summarizes several of these key studies, as well as some of the limitations and challenges of research in this field.

Ziguras and Stuart (2000) conducted a meta-analysis of forty-four case management research studies conducted during the past twenty years. The authors specifically focused on the effectiveness of case management services with individuals diagnosed with a mental illness. They compared outcomes of two predominant case management models: assertive community treatment (ACT) and clinical case management, and analyzed the effects on twelve outcome variables. Their results concluded that both types of case management were more effective than usual treatment in four outcome variables (family burden, family satisfaction with services, cost of care, and number of hospital days). In addition, the ACT model reduced total number of hospitalizations and the proportion of clients hospitalized. Overall, it appeared that the ACT model of case management had some demonstrable advantages over clinical case management in reducing hospitalizations.

Another study (Bedell, Cohen, and Sullivan, 2000) attempted to explore the effectiveness of different models of case management for persons with severe mental illness. The researchers classified previous studies by whether case managers directly provided services (full service), brokered them from other providers (broker), or combined these two approaches (hybrid). Eight outcome variables were identified (increased retention/compliance, reduced hospital days, increased quality of life, increased level of functioning, use of community services, reduced cost, reduced symptoms, and increased satisfaction) and eight published case management reviews were assessed to determine how the effectiveness of these different case management models varied. This study found that the full service model appeared to be most effective in impacting positive client outcomes, while the broker model raised serious questions regarding its effectiveness.

One of the challenges in researching case management effectiveness is the lack of an adequate sample to sufficiently conduct statistical analyses. Katz et al. (2000) addressed this issue by analyzing data collected through the HIV Cost and Services Utilization Study (HCSUS), in which 2,832 HIV-infected adults were surveyed. Need and unmet need for supportive services were assessed and how case management impacted unmet need in this national probability sample of HIV-infected adults. Benefits advocacy, housing, home health care, emotional counseling, and substance abuse treatment were identified as supportive services. Their overall finding was that

> after adjusting for potential confounders, participants who had contact with a case manager in the previous six months had less unmet need for all supportive services, and the effect was statistically significant for home health care, emotional counseling, and any unmet need. (Katz et al., 2000, p. 65)

In addition, it was found that greater intensity of case management services resulted in greater effectiveness; in other words, the more contact a client had with his or her case manager, the less he or she experienced an unmet need.

Rapp and Wintersteen (1989) reviewed the results of twelve demonstration projects that incorporated the strengths model of case management with severely mentally ill individuals in the state of Kansas. For the sake of consistency, each project implemented the same model, meaning that staffing qualifications and supervision, as well as specific case management activities were prescribed prior to service delivery. This strategy decreased the chance of comparing two or more *different* types of approaches, an issue which has been identified in the literature (Chamberlain and Rapp, 1991; Chernesky, 1999; Fleishman, 1998; Piette et al., 1995). The outcome indicators for this study were client goal achievement (measuring the number of treatment plan goals attained) and hospitalizations. Across the twelve sites, clients cumulatively accomplished 79 percent of their treatment plan goals, indicating a high level of achievement.

Clients enrolled in case management services provided by the twelve demonstration projects had fewer hospitalizations. In fact, they found that clients in eleven of the projects were hospitalized below the state average of hospitalizations for persons enrolled in community mental health support programs. An interesting finding was that the project whose clients had more hospitalizations than the state average was one in which case managers had a significant amount of client contact in the office, instead of in the community.

An outcome that has gained increased attention is how case management potentially prevents the provision of expensive medical care. A cost-effective study was performed in Florida to determine if the provision of case management and new drugs impacted the amount of Medicaid spent on persons with AIDS (Mitchell and Anderson, 2000). Medicaid and eligibility data from 1993 to 1997 were analyzed in the state of Florida to evaluate the effect of participation in the Medicaid waiver for persons with AIDS on monthly spending. Individuals enrolled in the Medicaid waiver are also provided case management services, compared to those who are not enrolled. The study found that overall monthly expenditures were higher for nonparticipants than for those enrolled in the waiver. In addition, inpatient spending was significantly higher for nonenrollees than for enrollees. The authors concluded that the AIDS case management component of the AIDS waiver program provided a continuity of care, as well as assistance with AIDS medication compliance. As a result, it appears that the use of these medications can reduce expensive inpatient hospital care, and case management may play an important role in this area.

Chernesky (1999) proposed that research on HIV/AIDS case management had failed to keep pace with the growth and development of the field. Thus, she reviewed relevant research in the literature to conceptualize it into a framework that would guide this area of research. Chernesky identified twenty-five research-based articles on HIV/AIDS case management published in professional journals, and classified them into four different categories: (1) client-level; (2) case- manager level; (3) case management programs or models; and (4) systems-level, particularly on regional or statewide approaches. A brief description of each research study and its findings was presented, organized by category.

Chernesky (1999) identified gaps in research in this field, including the lack of comparable research related to case management for persons with HIV/AIDS, and difficulty in identifying and agreeing upon outcome variables. Furthermore, research has focused on systems-level appraisals rather than outcomes for individual clients indicated that this has been in the format of program case studies, instead of comparison of case management models or a determination of how the availability of community resources effects case management. Paramount to the dilemmas in conducting HIV/AIDS case management research is the fact that there continues to be a lack of standardization of case management in this field. Being able to accurately describe the practice of HIV/AIDS case management has become a research challenge in itself.

Clearly, several research design and ethical issues exist in the field of HIV/AIDS case management. Fleishman (1998, p. 27) identified four overriding issues that must be clearly defined when approaching this endeavor:

1. nature of case management intervention (gatekeeper versus broker);
2. training and qualifications of case managers;
3. characteristics of clients or target population; and
4. outcomes to be affected, whether it is utilization of resources, health status of client, or cost effectiveness of program.

Other issues must also be addressed in this arena. One is the sample size in the research study and whether it is sufficient to generalize findings. Another is related to the number of case managers employed in the study; for example, if there is only one case manager, the results of the study could be due to personal characteristics of the case manager and not necessarily due to the intervention. Setting is another issue, for as the service provision in this field has grown during the past twenty years, models with unique characteristics have emerged depending upon the setting in which case management is delivered. For instance, in a medical setting, case management activities and qualifications of the case management team may look very different from case management services delivered in a community-based setting.

Systems also have an impact on the effectiveness of case management services. The model of case management is a true embodiment of the social work value "person in environment" and these activities cannot be carried out in a vacuum. However, if a system is fragmented, it results in the inability to effectively serve individuals with certain needs, and the case manager's capability to link clients to care and accomplish goals outlined in the treatment plan will ultimately fail.

Another issue related to systems-level capacity is when a client may be utilizing services from several different providers, each with its own case management team. As a result, the client may be case managed by individuals in several programs, which may also employ different approaches or interventions. Thus, a client may receive an "extra dose" of case management. The challenge for the researcher is to determine the best possible method to single out the effects of the specific case management model being researched.

EMERGING ISSUES IN THE FIELD

As the HIV/AIDS epidemic continues to affect various populations, in addition to the promising treatments and availability of treatments, the manner in which case management services are delivered will continue to be transformed. This is an opportunity for the field of social work to provide leadership in research and practice efforts, and influence how research findings will be translated into the practice field.

A recent qualitative study by Merithew and Davis-Satterla (2000) identified how case management has changed due to the advent of protease inhibitors. Forty interviews were conducted with executive directors, supervisors, and case managers to determine the AIDS case management model under which five AIDS service organizations practice. Their findings included the identification of two distinct streams of clients: those who were experiencing a positive improvement in their health and their lessening need to rely on case management, and those whose HIV was exacerbated by other coexisting factors, including substance use, mental illness, and/or a lack of living skills. This second group continued to require an intense level of case management. Some of the concerns regarding this emerging population are related to how this would effect case managers' abilities to manage a caseload of clients which may be more complex and require more time to address their multiple issues and needs.

Issues related to returning to work are also a growing concern for clients, whose health may now be improving to a point where this is a viable option. Thus, case managers should be familiar with benefits and how returning to work may affect a client's continued receipt of benefits (particularly health insurance). In addition, clients' concerns regarding job discrimination and whether their health will continue to allow them to work requires case managers to address these issues.

The introduction of protease inhibitors has also impacted case management because of the need to focus on treatment adherence issues. Individuals who do not comply with the prescribed treatment regimen jeopardize the effectiveness of these drugs, and consequently, their own health. Various interventions have been developed and adopted by providers to support patients in their attempt to follow a complicated regime of multiple pills, dosage requirements, and side effects. Some of these interventions include increased health education provided at the time of initiating the drugs, as well as throughout treatment; pill boxes with weekly dosages organized by day and time; and pagers allow individuals to be beeped and reminded of dosages.

Case managers' activities have also been affected by these new treatments. In a study conducted by Merithew and Davis-Satterla (2000), case managers identified that their relationships with primary medical providers have been strengthened to address treatment adherence issues with a team approach. In addition, case managers have increasingly been placed in an educator role, requiring that they remain updated on the latest available medications and their side effects. Finally, case managers continue to problem solve and remove barriers for their clients as they face physical and emotional challenges to adhering with their treatment.

SERVICE IMPLICATIONS

After twenty years of delivering services to persons living with HIV/AIDS, case management continues to be a critical component in the field of social work. However, it appears that little consensus regarding the definition and practice standards has been made among experts in this field. Despite this, organizations continue to implement and financially support the delivery of case management services. In summary, several of the key issues that case managers who work in the field of HIV/AIDS face are:

- With the advent of new therapies, clients are long-term survivors, creating a shift in the focus of service needs of clients.
- Concurrently, since many of these treatment regimens are complicated, case managers are expected to address treatment adherence issues as a component of their case management duties.
- As the rates of HIV infection continue to increase in different communities, including impoverished families, substance users, the chronically mentally ill, and persons of color, the ability to adequately coordinate clients' service needs becomes more challenging and complex.
- With an increase in the number of individuals becoming HIV positive, as well as longer survival rates, case managers are expected to maintain larger caseload sizes. Subsequently, this also requires increased paperwork and reporting standards, which in turn impact the amount of time available for staff to engage and develop trusting relationships with their clients.
- Since the level of allocated resources has not correlated with the increase in the number of HIV-positive individuals, case managers frequently find themselves in a brokering or gatekeeper role. Again, particularly for practitioners who have an interest in developing their clinical and advocacy skills, this may result in feelings of frustration and preliminary burnout.
- Case managers' abilities to effectively deliver services are impacted by the service delivery system in which they operate. When there is a lack of service providers or poor coordination among other service agencies, case managers are required to utilize different abilities, including negotiating skills and community development to successfully coordinate clients' service needs.

To address some of these issues, the following recommendations may be made:

- Provide intensive orientation training, as well as ongoing training opportunities, which need to be integrated for optimal case management performance. Furthermore, as the medical research field continues to identify new medications to treat HIV disease, case managers must remain abreast of these medications, their side effects, and how they impact patients' quality of life.

- Provide supportive supervision for case managers on a regular and consistent basis. During supervision, case managers may have the opportunity to receive ongoing feedback and direction regarding their work activities. In addition, supervision can provide a forum in which case managers may identify the need for training and skills building, as well as receive emotional support that may prevent burnout.

- Similarly, provide a supportive organizational environment, which could include flexible work hours, mental health days, and staff appreciation activities. When possible, the implementation of team-based models of case management may impact both staff performance and the quality of services received by clients.

- Implement and monitor standards of care to ensure that case management services are consistent across populations and among staff.

CONCLUSION

After twenty years of developing and providing medical and social services for persons living with HIV/AIDS, the need for continually identifying effective service delivery models is necessary. This disease has changed dramatically during the past two decades, affecting diverse populations that have faced complex cultural, social, and economic barriers to receiving adequate care. In addition, as new treatments have been discovered and prescribed for HIV-infected individuals, the approach to providing services that continually address the psychosocial needs of this population must also change. This beckons a continued partnership between practitioners and researchers, providing the forum to persistently assess how this epidemic impacts the practice models and conversely, how the delivery of effective services impacts the psychosocial and medical needs of persons living with HIV. Without a doubt, there is a persistent need for continued research of case management services for persons with special health care needs. Specific issues that continue to impact the delivery of services related to case management include caseload size, use of a team approach versus an individual case manager, expected duration of case management services, and specific activities to be included in case management models.

REFERENCES

Austin, C. D. (1993). Case management: A systems perspective. *Families in Society: The Journal of Contemporary Human Services, 74*(8), 453-459.

Austin, C. D., Low, J., Roberts, E. A., and O'Connor, K. (1985). *Case management: A critical review.* Seattle: Pacific Northwest Long Term Care Gerontology Center, University of Washington.

Bedell, J. R., Cohen, N. L., and Sullivan, A. (2000). Case management: The current best practices and the next generation of innovation. *Community Mental Health Journal, 36*(2), 179-194.

Chamberlain, R. and Rapp, C. A. (1991). A decade of case management: A methodological review of outcome research. *Community Mental Health Journal, 27*(3), 171-188.

Chernesky, R. H. (1999). A review of HIV/AIDS case management research. *Journal of Case Management, 8*(2), 105-113.

Chernesky, R. H. and Grube, B. (2000). Examining the HIV/AIDS case management process. *Health and Social Work, 25*(4), 243-253.

Emlet, C. A., and Guaz, S. S. (1998). Service use patterns in HIV/AIDS case management: A five-year study. *Journal of Case Management, 7*(1), 3-9.

Fleishman, J. A. (1998). Research design issues in evaluating the outcomes of case management for persons with HIV. In H. A. B. Health Resources and Services Administration (Ed.), *Evaluating HIV case management: Invited research and evaluation papers* (pp. 25-50). Rockville, MD: Government Printing Office.

Harris, M. and Bergman, H. C. (1987). Case management with the chronically mentally ill: A clinical perspective. *American Journal of Orthopsychiatry, 57*(2), 296-302.

Indyk, D., Belville, R., Lachapelle, S., Gordon, G., and Dewart, T. (1993). A community-based approach to HIV case management: Systematizing the unmanageable. *Social Work, 38,* 380-387.

Katz, M. H., Cunningham, W. E., Mor, V., Andersen, R. M., Kellogg, T., Zierler, S., Crystal, S. C., Stein, M. D., Cylar, K., Bozzette, S. A., et al. (2000). Prevalence and predictors of unmet need for supportive services among HIV-infected persons: Impact of case management. *Medical Care, 38*(1), 58-69.

Littrell, E. (1998). HIV case managers: The challenge and the responsibility. In H. A. B. Health Resources and Services Administration (Ed.), *Evaluating HIV* case management: Invited research and evaluation papers (pp. 189-216). Rockville, MD: Government Printing Office.

Merithew, M. A. and Davis-Satterla, L. (2000). Protease inhibitors: Changing the way AIDS case management does business. *Qualitative Health Research, 10*(5), 632-645.

Mitchell, J. M. and Anderson, K. H. (2000). Effects of case management and new drugs on Medicaid AIDS spending. *Health Affairs, 19*(4), 234-243.

Moore, S. (1992). Case management and the integration of services: How service delivery systems shape case management. *Social Work, 37*(5), 418-423.

NASW (1992). *NASW standards for social work case management.* Washington, DC: National Association of Social Workers.

Netting, F. E. (1992). Case management: Service or symptom? *Social Work, 37*(2), 160-164.

O'Connor, G. G. (1988). Case management: System and practice. *Social Casework: The Journal of Contemporary Social Work, 69,* 97-106.

Pescosolido, B. A., Wright, E. R., and Sullivan, W. P. (1995). Communities of care: A theoretical perspective on case management models in mental health. *Advances in Medical Sociology, 6,* 37-79.

Piette, J., Fleishman, J. A., Mor, V., and Thompson, B. (1992). The structure and process of AIDS case management. *Health and Social Work, 17*(1), 47-56.

Piette, J. D., Thompson, B. J., Fleishman, J. A., and Vincent, M. (1995). The organization and delivery of AIDS case management. In V. J. Lynch, G. A. Lloyd, and M. F. Fimbres (Eds.), *The changing face of AIDS: Implications for social work practice* (Second edition) (pp. 39-62). Westport, CT: Auburn House.

Raiff, N. R. and Shore, B. K. (1993). *Advanced case management: New strategies for the nineties* (Volume 66). Newbury Park, NJ: Sage Publications.

Rapp, C. A. and Wintersteen, R. (1989). The strengths model of case management: Results from twelve demonstrations. *Psychosocial Rehabilitation Journal, 13*(1), 23-32.

Rose, S. M. and Moore, V. L. (1995). Case management. In R. L. Edwards (Ed.), *Encyclopedia of social work* (Nineteenth edition). Washington, DC: NASW Press.

Rothman, J. (1994). *Practice with highly vulnerable clients: Case management and community-based service.* Englewood Cliffs, NJ: Prentice-Hall.

Sowell, R. L. and Grier, J. (1995). Integrated case management: The AID Atlanta model. *Journal of Case Management, 4,* 15-21.

Stein, L. I. and Test, M. A. (1980). An alternative to mental hospital treatment. I: Conceptual model, treatment program, and clinical evaluation. *Archives of General Psychiatry, 37,* 392-397.

Vourlekis, B. (1992). The policy and professional context of case management practice. In B. S. Vourlekis and R. R. Greene (Eds.), *Social work case management* (pp. 1-10). New York: Aldine de Gruyter.

Weil, M. and Karls, J. M. (1985). *Case management in human service practice.* San Francisco: Jossey-Bass.

Ziguras, S. J. and Stuart, G. W. (2000). A meta-analysis of the effectiveness of mental health case management over 20 years. *Psychiatric Services, 51*(11), 1410-1421.

Chapter 3

The Transtheoretical Model of Behavior and Injection Drug Use

San Patten

INTRODUCTION

The sharing of injection equipment among injection drug users (IDUs) is the second most common mode of HIV transmission next to sexual contact. The transmission of HIV can be prevented by changing high-risk behaviors such as unprotected sex and sharing used injection equipment. One of the primary modes for HIV transmission through drug injection is the use of HIV-contaminated syringes, needles, vials, spoons, filters, and other such equipment. HIV infection is highly preventable, and short of a cure for AIDS or immunization for HIV, the most important action charged to health and social service professionals is to eliminate the behaviors that make the spread of HIV possible.

The challenge for health and social service professionals is to promote healthy behavior changes even among individuals who have no desire or intention to change. Prochaska's transtheoretical model of behavior change, also known as the stages of change model, integrates several psychotherapy theories or models into one comprehensive framework for explaining the underlying structure of behavior change (Prochaska and Velicer, 1997). The transtheoretical model

I would like to thank Drs. Ardene Vollman and Billie Thurston for their guidance and support; Krista McLuskey for her expert editing; Barb LeMarchand-Unich, Calgary Regional Health Authority—Family Planning Clinic; Jo Wood, Calgary Regional Health Authority—Safeworks Calgary; Allan Clear, Harm Reduction Coalition, New York; Stacey Rubin, Streetwork Project, New York; Garth Goertz, AIDS Calgary Awareness Association; and Guy Milner, Calgary Regional Health Authority—Southern Alberta HIV/AIDS Clinic.

(TTM) contributes to existing psychotherapy approaches by accounting for individuals who are not ready to make active changes in their behaviors. Other behavior change models have significant failure rates because they attempt to enact change in people who are either resistant to change or do not see their behavior as problematic. The majority of people engaging in high-risk behaviors are not prepared for action and will not be served by traditional action-oriented prevention programs. Health promotion can have a much greater impact if it shifts from an action paradigm to a stage paradigm (Prochaska and Velicer, 1997).

The TTM was initially developed for smoking cessation but its application has rapidly expanded to include investigations and applications with a broad range of physical and mental health behaviors. These include alcohol and substance abuse, anxiety and panic disorders, delinquency, eating disorders and obesity, high-fat diets, mammography screening, medication compliance, unplanned pregnancy prevention, pregnancy and smoking, sedentary lifestyles, gambling addiction, and sun exposure (Prochaska and Velicer, 1997).

Three studies were identified that related the TTM to the behaviors of IDUs. The AIDS Community Demonstration Projects Research Group studied a community-level intervention based on the TTM (Jamner, Wolitski, and Corby, 1997). The intervention aimed to modify attitudes and beliefs about prevention methods among the community members by providing models of successful risk-reduction strategies adopted by members of the target population. The intervention featured role model stories developed from the real-life experiences of local community members. These stories depicted members of the target population moving from earlier to later stages of change. The TTM was applied as an outcome measure to examine the impact of an educational intervention directed at IDUs targeting condom use and bleach use to clean drug paraphernalia (Jamner, Wolitski, and Corby, 1997).

The two other studies applying the TTM to IDUs were restricted to drug rehabilitation and condom use (Bowen and Trotter, 1995; Prochaska et al., 1994). The TTM is well suited to the IDU population because it recognizes that chronic behavior patterns are usually under some combination of biological, social, and self-control. Also, stage-matched interventions have been primarily designed to enhance self-controls, rather than therapist controls, which are not conducive to illicit behavior such as injection drug use.

The objective of this chapter is to examine the utility of the TTM for promoting reduction of needle use risk behaviors among IDUs as a means to prevent HIV transmission. This chapter will outline:

1. the challenges of applying the TTM to IDU behaviors with respect to HIV prevention;
2. the four major components of the TTM (stages of change, processes of change, decisional balance, and self-efficacy) as they relate to IDUs;
3. how health and social service practitioners are currently using the TTM; and
4. current and future research using the TTM for IDUs as a target population.

RISK REDUCTION AMONG IDUS

In attempting to apply the TTM to behaviors that place IDUs at high risk of becoming infected with HIV, it is important to understand the nature of the behaviors and the nature of the risks involved with injection drug use. The nature and multitude of the high-risk behaviors among IDUs poses many challenges to health and social service practitioners who try to encourage HIV risk reduction. Sexual behaviors, such as unprotected sex and having multiple partners, pose significant HIV risk to IDUs, especially as a result of the heightened sexual activity that coincides with the use of drugs such as cocaine (Springer, 1991). The second domain of behaviors that should be targeted by risk-reduction efforts is injection practices that place IDUs at risk of a range of poor health outcomes, from collapsed veins and abscesses to HIV or hepatitis infection, or drug overdose. Needle-use behaviors such as reusing needles, poor vein care, sharing needles and other drug paraphernalia, and backloading are important but difficult to change. Backloading is a method used by IDUs to ensure that their hit will enter a vein. It involves pulling blood back into the syringe to mix with the drug. Needle sharing after practicing backloading is a primary means for blood contamination between IDUs. This chapter will focus on injection behaviors, rather than sexual behaviors, as the application of the TTM to condom use has been researched fairly extensively (Bowen and Trotter, 1995; Grimley et al., 1995; Jamner, Wolitski, and Corby, 1997).

The basic underlying principle of risk reduction concerning injection behaviors can be summarized by the following four messages directed at IDUs:

1. get off drugs;
2. if you cannot stop using drugs, stop injecting drugs;
3. if you cannot or will not stop injecting drugs, do not share needles (or other drug paraphernalia); and
4. if you cannot or will not stop sharing needles, at least disinfect needles between sharing partners using common household bleach (Watters et al., 1990).

Health and social service practitioners need to promote change at the level of risk reduction that is most amenable for each individual IDU. The behavior change goal of health promotion interventions will vary depending on where in the spectrum of risk reduction the IDU is willing to make changes. For example, if an IDU is unwilling to quit injection drug use, then it would be futile for a nurse to prescribe drug addiction treatment. However, that same IDU may be willing to change the way in which he or she injects drugs in order to prevent HIV infection; the nurse would then apply the TTM to design interventions that work toward an end goal of safer injection.

High-risk injection behaviors are difficult to change for many reasons, and they present significant challenges in the application of the TTM. The challenges are twofold. The first major challenge in applying the TTM to HIV risk reduction among IDUs is the nature of injection behaviors and the context within which they occur. Injection drug use is an illicit, underground, and therefore largely concealed activity, which makes it difficult for health and social service practitioners to access those who are most at risk of HIV infection. The addictive nature of injected drugs, such as morphine, heroin, and cocaine and the accompanying cravings and drug-induced psychoses also make risk-reduction efforts difficult. Cravings for a drug hit are extremely powerful for individuals who are addicted, and these cravings often override any attention to HIV risk, vein care, or overdose. The use of injection drugs is socially unacceptable and IDUs are naturally defensive against criticisms or suggestions for change that come from mainstream health and social service practitioners. Finally, injection drug use is highly ritualized and occurs within very specific social contexts and situations that are virtually unknown to health and social service practitioners. The challenge for health and social service practitioners is to adapt the principles of behavior change to the IDU population by taking into account the culturally specific contexts within which drug use occurs.

The second major challenge of applying the TTM to the IDU population is the nature of the risk of HIV infection itself. Behaviors such as smoking, high-fat diet, lack of exercise, and sun exposure have cumulative negative effects that build in severity over time. However, unlike such cumulative effects, HIV infection only requires one event to have its negative effect manifested. The fact that HIV infection does not require multiple and prolonged exposure to have adverse consequences brings a sense of immediacy to risk-reduction efforts. Risk of HIV infection varies with type of drug and/or frequency of injection. For example, cocaine users are at much higher risk of HIV infection. Due to the short-lived nature of the high, users must inject many consecutive hits in order to maintain the drug's effects. Cocaine produces fleeting drug euphoria, with the user often wanting the next injection within fifteen minutes. Thus, cocaine users will often binge, injecting almost continuously until the supply of the drug is exhausted, placing them at significant risk of HIV infection (Patten and Vollman, 1999). Other important risk factors include duration of drug use (new initiates into drug use tend to be more erratic and practice less risk reduction than do long-time users), social setting of drug use (injecting in shooting galleries places IDUs at much higher risk of HIV than injecting at home), and ethnic minority status (blacks and Hispanics are at higher risk for HIV). In order for health and social service practitioners to be successful, it is crucial that they consider these differences among IDUs and adjust interventions accordingly.

THE TRANSTHEORETICAL MODEL OF BEHAVIOR CHANGE

There are four main components to the TTM: (1) stages of change; (2) processes of change; (3) self-efficacy; and (4) motivation and decision making (DiClemente and Prochaska, 1992). This chapter explains each component of the TTM and apply the principles to HIV risk reduction by suggesting examples with IDUs.

Stages of Change

The first component of the TTM is the stages of change. The stages are a central organizing construct that describes *when* people are ready to change and *what* needs to be changed. The stages of change are the temporal dimension of the TTM that integrates processes and principles of change from different theories of intervention, hence the name *transtheoretical* (Prochaska and Velicer, 1997). One of the major contributions of the TTM to existing psychotherapy models is that it accounts for those individuals who are not ready to make active changes in their health-related behaviors. The TTM also contributes a dimension of time; change implies phenomena occurring over time, rather than a single discrete event, such as quitting smoking cold turkey. The TTM construes change as a process involving progress through a series of six stages:

1. precontemplation;
2. contemplation;
3. preparation;
4. action;
5. maintenance; and
6. termination.

The TTM's six stages of change are presented in Table 3.1, including a brief description of the characteristics of people who are in the stage, and an illustrative example of an IDU in each stage of change. The IDU in the examples has chosen to reduce his or her HIV risk by eliminating needle sharing.

Relapse, when an individual returns to a previous stage, unfortunately tends to be the rule when action is taken for most health-related problem behavior. Most people in action or maintenance do not regress all the way back to precontemplation. However, an IDU may if he or she feels like a failure, embarrassed, ashamed, and guilty. The IDU may become demoralized and resist thinking about changing injection behaviors. As a result, he or she can return to and remain in the precontemplation stage for an indeterminate period of time. Most

TABLE 3.1. Stages of Change in the Transtheoretical Model

Stage of Change	Characteristics	Example
Precontemplation (PC)	Engages in risk behavior. Has no intention of changing within the next six months. May be uninformed, in denial, or demoralized from previous failures. Defensive and resistant to change, avoids addressing risky behavior.	An IDU in PC does not think about used needles and sees no risk in their use, believing that no friends have HIV. Friends and family see the IDU's behaviors as dangerous and pressure IDU to change injection habits, but the IDU becomes defensive and denies the problem.
Contemplation (C)	Engages in risky behavior but is aware of problem. Seriously considering change within six months, but has not yet made a commitment to take action. Indecisive, lacks commitment to enact significant change in high-risk behaviors.	An IDU in C realizes that sharing needles places oneself at risk, but fears insulting friends by refusing to share with them. The IDU begins to seek information and alternatives to high-risk behavior. He or she is aware of the risks involved and knows that high-risk behaviors should be changed but is not yet ready to do so.
Preparation (P)	Still engages in high-risk behavior, but intends to take action within the next month. Has typically taken some significant action in the past year. Is on the verge of taking action and needs to set goals.	An IDU in P will have to set an end goal somewhere along the risk reduction continuum and make firm commitments with strict criteria such as, "I will use a new needle for every hit of drug." He or she has inquired about the needle exchange program and is considering using it.
Action (A)	Has modified the behavior, experiences, or environment within the last six months. Involves overt behavioral changes and requires considerable commitment of time and energy.	The IDU in A has begun to use one new needle for every hit of drug. The IDU may encounter pitfalls that may be external (situational or social) or internal (emotional or psychological) in origin. It will be much easier to abstain from sharing if friends make the same effort.

TABLE 3.1 *(continued)*

Stage of Change	Characteristics	Example
Maintenance (M)	Works to prevent relapse and consolidate the gains attained during action. Is less tempted to relapse and has become increasingly more confident to continue changes. A continuation, not an absence of change.	The IDU has used a new needle for every hit of drug in the last six months and is using coping strategies for high-risk situations. Needle sharing may be triggered if the environment is filled with negative cues, for example, in a shooting gallery. The IDU still makes a conscious effort to continue HIV risk reduction such as purposefully avoiding shooting galleries.
Termination (T)	Feels zero temptation and complete confidence. New, healthier behavior has become second nature. This stage is unlikely for most addictive behaviors.	An IDU will always be faced with situations in which needle sharing is a temptation, and as long as he or she is using injection drugs, will have to actively maintain new needle use behaviors.

people regress only to the contemplation or preparation stages, when they begin to consider plans for their next action attempt while trying to learn from their recent efforts. For example, an IDU may have relapsed back to needle sharing while at a party with friends who passed prepared shots in needles. The IDU must again set firm goals against needle sharing and learn to avoid social settings involving the temptation to take someone else's needle.

Processes of Change

The stages of change represent a temporal dimension that describes *when* particular shifts in attitudes, intentions, and behaviors occur. The processes of change are a second major dimension of the TTM that explains *how* these shifts occur (Prochaska, DiClemente, and Norcross, 1992). The ten processes of change are the covert and overt activities that people use to progress through the stages (Prochaska and Velicer, 1997). Processes of change provide important tools for intervention programs, since the processes are like the independent variables that people need to apply to move from one stage to the next. Table 3.2 presents a summary of the various processes of change and provides illustrative examples of how an IDU may progress through each process.

The TTM integrates the models from several psychotherapy approaches as processes that have priority at various stages. In the early stages, people apply cognitive, affective, and evaluative processes to progress through the stages (Prochaska and Velicer, 1997). Experiential processes are important in helping the individual change thoughts, feelings, and attitudes related to problem behaviors. During action and maintenance, behavioral-type processes are most predominant, such as conditioning, commitments, contingencies, environmental controls, and social support. Behavioral processes are central to individuals changing behaviors and relationships. Helping relationships, consciousness raising, and self-liberation are the three processes used most frequently across twelve problem behaviors, whereas contingency management and stimulus control are the least commonly used processes (Prochaska and Norcross, 1994).

Self-Efficacy

Self-efficacy is the situation-specific confidence people have that helps them cope with high-risk situations without relapsing to their unhealthy or high-risk habit. In order to change, individuals must be confident that they can abstain from, avoid, reduce, or control the problem behavior despite being faced with temptations in the surrounding environment or situations. Efficacy scores (using Janis and Mann's [1997] Decision Making Model) vary significantly with precontemplators having the lowest level of self-efficacy, and maintainers, the highest (Prochaska et al., 1994). Temptation reflects the intensity of urges to engage in a specific habit when in the midst of difficult situations. The most common types of tempting situations are negative effect or emotional distress, positive social situations, and cravings (Prochaska and Velicer, 1997). Efficacy and temptation interact across the stages of change; efficacy rises as temptation falls. As an IDU progresses from precontemplation through to action, he or she is better able to resist temptations such as prepared syringes available at a social gathering or a used needle offered by a friend.

TABLE 3.2. Processes of Change of the Transtheoretical Model

Process of Change	Characteristics	Example
Consciousness raising	Individuals need to raise their awareness of the negative consequences of their behavior.	An IDU in precontemplation will have to be convinced that HIV infection is a real threat, that alternatives exist to needle sharing, and important ways in which injection practices can be modified to prevent HIV infection.
Dramatic relief	Individuals need to release and express emotions related to their high-risk behavior. Life events, such as the death of a close friend or family member, can move people into contemplation emotionally, especially if the death was related to the high-risk behavior.	IDUs who are suffering from depression or abuse may feel that HIV infection is the least of their worries, but need to accept that they are able to change high-risk behaviors. If an IDU knows that a friend died of AIDS because of a contaminated needle, grief may be a powerful motivator for changing personal injection practices.
Environmental reevaluation	In precontemplation, individuals need to recognize how the presence or absence of a personal habit affects one's social environment.	IDUs need to acknowledge the effect that needle sharing could have on people close to them, that is: What if I became HIV positive and passed it on to my partner? IDUs may see themselves as role models for others, such as for new initiates into injection drug use.
Self-reevaluation	This process is most important when individuals are moving from contemplation to preparation, when people assess how they feel and think about the behavior. People may become aware of their guilt about a particular behavior.	An IDU needs to decide on priorities and which values to act on. He or she must also decide if it is more important to get a quick high and share drugs with friends or to practice safe injection and avoid HIV infection.
Self-liberation	While preparing for action, individuals become self-liberated, that is, believe that they can change and make the commitment to act on that belief.	For an IDU this means asserting control over selected injection behaviors, telling oneself that he or she is able to practice safer injection, and making a firm decision to do so.

Process of Change	Characteristics	Example
Reinforcement management	During action, individuals need to provide consequences for taking steps in a particular direction, including the use of punishments for slips, or rewards for making positive changes.	The rewards IDUs choose for succeeding in HIV risk reduction may include more or larger hits of their drug of choice, alcohol, or cigarettes; these rewards may be considered as health damaging.
Helping relationships	Helping relationships can include those with health professionals who are actively involved in assisting the person to change or supportive members of a social network.	It is important for individuals making stressful changes to have someone with whom they can be open and trusting about their problems. An IDU may be much more willing to change if a significant other provides instrumental support, such as by exchanging needles.
Counterconditioning	During the action and maintenance stages, individuals need to substitute healthier behaviors for the high-risk behaviors.	IDUs need to learn how to use assertion to counter peer pressure in high-risk situations where they may be tempted to revert to needle sharing.
Stimulus control	People in action or maintenance need to remove stimuli that were associated with the unhealthy behavior, and add stimuli that signal the new behavior.	An IDU may ensure that used needles are not visible and tempting by ensuring that hazardous waste containers are placed around the house for rapid and easy disposal of used needles.
Social liberation	Social liberation requires an increase in social opportunities or alternatives, especially for people who are relatively deprived or oppressed.	Advocacy, empowerment programs, and appropriate policies can produce increased opportunities for HIV prevention among IDUs. Needle exchange programs are an important way to encourage IDUs not to share needles.

Motivation and Decision Making

Motivation describes the individual's reasons for wanting to change and the strength of commitment to make the changes. Decision making involves balancing the pros, or the benefits of changing the behavior, with the cons, or the costs of changing the behavior. Motivation and decision making are important constructs during the pre-action stages (precontemplation, contemplation, and preparation). An individual who progresses from precontemplation through to action must overcome the cons of change and increasingly recognize the pros, until the pros are higher than the cons. At this point, the individual is ready to make active changes in behavior. For example, with respect to trying to stop needle sharing, an IDU must place the pro of HIV prevention above the con of insulting friends by refusing to share their needles.

PRACTITIONERS' APPLICATIONS OF THE TTM

Health and social services practitioners who work with IDUs in the field of risk reduction (from drug treatment to vein care) include nurses, doctors, educators, social workers, counselors, and outreach workers. To assess how the TTM is used on a practical level by health and social work professionals, several key informants were interviewed who are either experts on the TTM and have applied the model to various other populations and behaviors, or who are experts on the IDU population and the specific challenges inherent with their high-risk behaviors.

The author acted as a participant observer in a focus group of health and social service practitioners who were developing a modified, user-friendlier version of the TTM as an interactive board game with clients. The participants of the focus group came from a variety of health and social services, and thus were experienced in a range of behavior change contexts. The health and social service practitioners involved had all used the TTM as a means of placing clients along the continuum of stages to customize interventions that would be appropriate for each client. The health and social service practitioners had experienced varying degrees of success with the model, but all agreed that TTM had excellent intuitive appeal and that it made sense. The focus group also agreed that the TTM needs to be modified to reduce the jargon to make it more accessible so that clients could monitor their own progress through the stages. In conceptualizing the various components, the health and social service practitioners found phrases embodying the stage or process helpful. Precontemplators, for example, may commonly use statements such as, "Yeah, but?" (rationalization of problem behavior), "You're the one with a problem" (denial of a problem behavior), or "I'll never be able to change" (futility in attempting to change). Most of the focus group participants were from academic backgrounds and were comfortable applying models and theories, in general. Thus, they were receptive to the idea of applying the TTM to HIV risk reduction among IDUs.

The other group, however, was less comfortable with the TTM. The author attended a staff meeting of the nurses and administrators of a local needle exchange program. The nurses all expressed familiarity with the TTM, but did not find it useful on a practical level. In particular, the nurses were very unlikely to talk to a client and think to themselves: this person is obviously in precontemplation. However, the needle exchange nurses did agree that the TTM makes sense and they agreed with its premises. They were resistant to the jargon and technical nature of the constructs of the TTM, but did informally use the ideas behind the TTM to personalize interventions with individual IDUs who are clients of the needle exchange program. One nurse stated that familiarity with the concepts behind the TTM allowed her to be sensitive to the readiness of clients to enact change, whether it be in injection behaviors or amount of drug consumption. This sensitivity, in turn, allowed the nurse to customize interactions with needle exchange clients so that her encouragement was appropriately and effectively targeted at behaviors, which are conducive to change for the better.

The Harm Reduction Coalition uses the TTM as a framework for the training curriculum of outreach workers and educators who work with IDUs. Harm reduction is a health promotion philosophy that has as its first priority a decrease in the negative consequences of drug use. Harm reduction tries to reduce problems associated with the drug use and recognizes that abstinence is not the only acceptable or important goal. For example, if an IDU seemed particularly resistant to drug treatment and had no intention to try to quit his or her drug use (i.e., the client was in precontemplation), the nurses would refrain from encouraging drug treatment, and focus on other behaviors, such as HIV prevention. Therefore, the TTM is used as a framework for the risk-reduction principles. Depending on the priorities and readiness of the IDU to act at various levels of risk reduction, the health and social service practitioners promote behavior change accordingly.

A nurse at the local needle exchange program periodically uses the model but does not find it especially useful. The nurse uses the model mostly as a diagnostic tool, as a gauge to assess where a client is. She assumes that a new client is at precontemplation and then lets the client demonstrate that he or she is at a higher level. Rather than try to haul, coerce, or pull people up the spiral, the nurse assumes the lowest stage and then lets the client demonstrate otherwise. Once the client has identified himself or herself as being at a certain stage, the nurse makes suggestions for progression to higher stages. Ultimately, the client maintains control over his or her behavior change. The nurse expressed that she does not use the model regularly. For her, the model's use is limited to identifying a client's stage but does not help her understand when and how to get someone from one stage to the next: "It's just a diagnostic model. It has no intrinsic engine that moves it along."

The author met with the manager of a local family planning clinic where they have operationalized the TTM for promotion of condom use to protect against STDs. The nurses at the clinic use the TTM to stage patients and have specified interventions, such as counseling and educational materials, that correspond with each stage. In each patient interview room, there is a guide for the nurses that lists staging questions, charting instructions, transition tips for discussing previous visits to the clinic, and descriptions of each stage. The nurses keep a running record of progression through the stages within the patients' medical records so that the patients' progress can be monitored and reinforced from visit to visit. The nurses use staging questions to place the patients within one of the five stages and have specific counseling interventions based upon the appropriate process of change to be used at each stage. The guide suggests questions to stimulate discussion with patients according to their stage. The nurse, for example, would ask a patient in the preparation stage of condom use the following questions: What do you see as being the next steps in starting to use condoms? How will you know when you're ready to start? When will you begin? What do you need to do to make this change happen? There are also specific pamphlets, brochures, videos, and supplies to present to patients at each stage of change that help a patient progress to the next stage of behavior change.

The author followed up with the clinic manager approximately two years after the initial introduction of the TTM guide for promoting condom use for protection against STDs. The manager of the family planning clinic stated that the nurses had moved to a more solution-focused case management strategy in which patients are asked to suggest their own solutions for adopting consistent condom use behaviors. One of the barriers experienced in the use of the TTM model for condom use was that the behavior is not dependent solely upon the readiness, decisions, and actions of the patient. Rather, the sexual partner of the patient must also be willing and ready to use condoms, a behavior that the nurses are not able to directly affect. The guide continues to act as a counseling trigger for the clinic nurses, however, and the nurses have continued to track the progress of clients through the stages in their medical charts. The patients' progression through the stages has not yet been evaluated, as the charts haven't been tabulated. This is an interesting area for further exploration for the family planning clinic, and may be an excellent source of evaluative data for the utility of the TTM.

The author also met with two social workers, one working in an AIDS service organization and one working in the local HIV/AIDS treatment clinic. Both social workers had an understanding of and experience with the TTM. The social worker from the AIDS service organization stated that he has applied the TTM to a range of behaviors in addition to addictions and HIV risk reduction. The TTM has been useful in working with clients who are in crisis situations, such as financial difficulty or domestic abuse. He stated that the TTM is useful in setting long-term goals and developing case plans for clients. He appreciated that the TTM does not use labels to classify individuals according to their compliance to enact desired behavior changes, but that it focuses on clients' readiness to change. The social worker finds that the TTM has helped him understand precontemplation as a precursor to active change efforts, and has developed an informal protocol for providing information to clients who may not have the motivation or knowledge necessary to begin changing their behaviors. One hurdle in applying the TTM is that many client contacts are one time only, making long-term follow-up and progression through the stages impossible. The social worker believes that the TTM is useful in identifying characteristics of people in various stages of change, but lacks concrete techniques of how to move people through the stages.

The social worker from the local HIV/AIDS treatment clinic has successfully incorporated the TTM into his everyday work with patients. He specifically applies the TTM for intake of new patients who may not be ready or willing to begin a rigorous regimen of HIV therapy. HIV-positive patients need to be ready and committed to take the medications to ensure successful treatment. Lack of adherence to drug regimens for HIV treatment can have detrimental effects on the patient, such as developing viral resistance to the drugs. The fact that patients have shown up at the clinic means that they have moved beyond precontemplation and are in contemplation about HIV treatment. The social worker spends time with patients to provide information about the drug regimens, strengthen their resolve to start HIV treatment, and work through the barriers to starting HIV treatment.

The social worker from the HIV/AIDS treatment clinic also applies the TTM, using a risk reduction framework, with patients who have addictions (usually alcohol, heroin, and cocaine). He explained that he understands that many patients are in precontemplation with regard to drug or alcohol abstinence, so he uses the TTM to move patients through the stages with regard to moderation of drug or alcohol use. This social worker said that, in general, the TTM helps him to be gentle and patient when dealing with addiction issues, and to understand that there is a natural cycle that patients must experience. The TTM helps him to "keep judgments in check" and to understand that patients "will get there eventually," usually within two years. Although the social worker applies the TTM's early stages (precontemplation, contemplation, preparation) fairly regularly, he has less experience actualizing the later stages (action, maintenance, termination). With patients who have addictions, his work generally stops at preparation when he refers the patient to a drug treatment center and he loses contact with patients after they have progressed through to active behavior change. Such is the nature of the helping professions!

To be effectively implemented by health and social service practitioners in their efforts to reduce HIV transmission among IDUs, the TTM should be customized in the following ways:

1. translation of theoretical jargon and constructs into "real-life" examples and scenarios that are culturally and linguistically appropriate;
2. use the TTM as a framework for moving clients or patients along the harm reduction continuum;
3. for ongoing contacts with clients or patients, document their progression through the stages for effective follow-up;

4. create behavior-specific interventions, queries, and cues for each stage and process of change; and
5. use the TTM to set long-term goals for individuals.

The TTM does not intrinsically suggest appropriate interventions for individuals in each stage. Rather, it suggests only general strategies and approaches for health and social service practitioners to use when counseling clients or patients. However, the trick is to understand which issues are common enough across various stages of change for a behavior such as needle sharing, so that they can be addressed in generic educational materials. The utility of the TTM for IDUs would be greatly improved by having specific learning materials and activities assigned for each stage and each behavior along the risk reduction continuum, much as the family planning clinic has for condom use. The design of a customized stage-appropriate curriculum will depend on several factors such as type of injection drug being used, ethnicity and cultural background of the IDU, education level, social norms, and so forth. In one ethnographic study of the social context of HIV risk reduction behaviors among IDUs, a series of four vignettes were developed describing specific social situations and settings in which high-risk injection drug use occurs (Patten and Vollman, 1999). This ethnography provides health and social service practitioners with an understanding of the complete psychosocial context surrounding the IDU and his or her behavior. Such an understanding is essential for a TTM practitioner in designing a customized set of interventions.

CURRENT AND FUTURE RESEARCH OF THE TTM WITH IDUs

Service providers who work with IDUs in HIV prevention may find the TTM useful in customizing their interactions with various clients. A health or social work practitioner speaking with IDUs who are not clients of the needle exchange program may find that they are in a precontemplative stage with respect to avoiding needle sharing. On the other hand, IDUs who have been clients of the needle exchange program for years may be in the maintenance stage of changing to safer injection behaviors. By staging each IDU that they work with, health and social service practitioners can gain a more in-depth understanding of his or her motivations. Health and social service practitioners can also use the staging to assess which social or environmental processes may be affecting the IDU at the time. For example, an IDU who is in the action phase of behavior change with respect to HIV risk reduction may have social influences such as helping relationships or counterconditioning.

Ethnographic studies of the social context of IDUs could be applied to intervention materials that are framed by the TTM. The intervention used by the researchers in the AIDS Community Demonstration Project (Jamner, Wolitski, and Corby, 1997) was designed from information obtained through open-ended interviews with members of the local IDU population. The researchers were able to develop role model stories that depicted positive changes in the attitudes, social norms, intentions, and behaviors of local target population members. The role model stories, complete with illustrative photographs, detailed:

1. the role model's experience in the target community;
2. the factors that motivated or facilitated his or her behavior change;
3. the specific changes made in behavior, intention, or attitudes;
4. the barriers to change encountered and how these barriers were overcome; and
5. the positive reinforcement received (Jamner, Wolitski, and Corby, 1997).

The role model stories can be customized to correspond to the stage at which the majority of the target population lies. To target precontemplators, for example, it is especially important to combine educational materials (which could be ignored) with environmental manipulation, such as provision of needles, condoms, and bleach kits (Jamner, Wolitski, and Corby, 1997). TTM practitioners should research each IDU and gain an understanding of his or her psychosocial context before prescribing stage-specific interventions. For example, in-depth research would be needed to design a certain stage-appropriate intervention for a Hispanic morphine user who wishes to improve his injection behaviors, versus an intervention for an Aborigine cocaine user who wishes to quit her drug use altogether. Thoroughness in designing customized interventions would help health and social service practitioners ensure success in moving clients from one stage to the next.

Other fruitful applications of the TTM are in the field of evaluation of intervention programs (Jamner, Wolitski, and Corby, 1997). Stage of change can serve as a primary outcome measure in a longitudinal evaluation of the impact of the intervention on progress toward a specific behavior change, such as safer injection. For example, if the majority of individuals at whom the intervention is targeted progress from one stage to the next, the intervention may be deemed successful, even if one individual has not yet actively terminated the problem behavior. TTM has important implications for how we evaluate interventions; stage progression is a logical criterion for stage-based interventions.

To have the greatest effect, an intervention needs to reach as large a proportion of the population of interest as possible (Velicer et al., 1994). The TTM was initially conceptualized as a population-level behavior change model in that it can be used to design interventions that would be appropriate for the entire population of IDUs, rather than just a minority of individuals who are ready for change (Prochaska and Norcross, 1994). Because very few IDUs come into contact with health professionals or other practitioners of the TTM, behavior change programs need to shift from reactive recruitment, in which the program is advertised and practitioners react when people express interest, to proactive recruitments, in which practitioners reach out to interact with all potential participants (DiClemente and Prochaska, 1992). Ideally, future research would involve customizing the TTM so that it could be used for interventions with total populations (Bellingham, 1990). The TTM could be applied at a population level to assess what percentage of the population is ready for change (in contemplation or preparation) and what percentage of the population is not ready for change (in precontemplation). For example, peer-delivered education and motivation campaigns, if stage-appropriate, could move the target population in the intervention area along the stage-of-change continuum. Interventions can be designed that are appropriate for everyone, with highly individualized interventions. However, if health promoters are to match the needs of entire populations, they first need to know the stage distributions of specific high-risk behaviors. Exploring high-risk behaviors among injection drug user populations is a difficult research problem, due to the hidden nature of the behavior.

Disseminating intervention materials to IDUs is also a problem. North Americans rely primarily on the mass media, such as television or newspapers, rather than specialized publications to learn about AIDS (Ornstein, 1989). Most IDUs, however, do not rely on the mass media, but rather on their immediate friends. Therefore, it is important to use peers, sexual partners, family members, and drug dealers as sources of information for IDUs who have little or no contact with mainstream culture. Three of the common factors associated with behavior change among IDUs with respect to HIV risk reduction were: talking with drug-using friends about AIDS; talking with sexual partners about AIDS; and talking with family about AIDS. This finding suggests that effective risk reduction should be conceptualized as a social process rather than as the behavior of an isolated individual (Gold and Skinner, 1992).

Crofts et al. (1996) found that among young initiates of injection drug use, the most common sources of information were the media (64 percent), parents (26 percent), and peer education programs (10 percent). However, even though the major source of information for these young IDUs was the media, the most credible source was peers and peer workers. Accordingly, further development of peer education programs is a most desirable strategy (Crofts et al., 1996). Peers can act as natural helpers and be trained to use the TTM to promote risk reduction amongst other IDUs. The TTM has enough intuitive grounding to be used by peer educators who are not necessarily health or social service professionals. In fact, peer educators have familiarity with the social context of drug-injection lifestyles, and can therefore better customize the TTM to ensure that its constructs are applied effectively to HIV risk among IDUs.

The TTM can also be used as a guideline for designing HIV risk reduction interventions. In the stage paradigm, intervention programs are matched to each individual's stage of change. An intervention guided by the TTM would influence behavior through the dissemination of information, development of behavioral skills, and positive reinforcement of progress toward consistent risk reduction (Jamner, Wolitski, and Corby, 1997). Behavior change can be expected to occur as a result of multiple exposures to the intervention materials, repeated reinforcement of protective behavior from peers, and a shift in the social norm toward the support of HIV-preventive practices, combined with increased access to condoms, sterile needles, and bleaching kits.

CONCLUSION

The TTM presents an innovative approach to health promotion that emphasizes:

1. behavior change viewed as a progression through a series of stages;
2. matching the most relevant independent variables and the most appropriate dependent variables to particular stages of change;
3. designing health promotion interventions that meet the needs of the individual at each stage of change; and
4. maximizing impacts on entire populations at risk by employing proactive recruitment and stage-matched, interactive, and individualized interventions.

Based on interviews with health and social service practitioners, the TTM seems to have excellent intuitive appeal and is useful in their efforts to assist clients or patients to make healthier choices. Further research is needed on the other constructs of the model: processes of change, decisional balance, self-efficacy, and temptation. More in-depth exploration is also needed on the model as a whole, rather than focusing on the stages of change in isolation. More research is necessary to determine how the TTM can be applied to IDUs within a population level. Other areas, such as drug use and risk reduction, need further study. In other areas of health, the TTM has proven to be remarkably robust, but some modifications have been required to reflect the unique aspect of the problem area.

REFERENCES

Bellingham, R. (1990). Debunking the myth of individual health promotion. *Occupational Medicine, 5*(4), 665-675.

Bowen, A. M. and Trotter, R. II. (1995). HIV risk in intravenous drug users and crack cocaine smokers: Predicting stage of change for condom use. *Journal of Consulting and Clinical Psychology, 63*(2), 238-248.

Crofts, N., Louie, R., Rosenthal, D., and Jolley, D. (1996). The first hit: Circumstances surrounding initiation into injecting. *Addiction, 91*(8), 1187-1196.

DiClemente, C. C. and Prochaska, J. O. (1992). Stages of change in the modification of problem behaviors. *Progress in Behavior Modification, 28,* 183-218.

Gold, R. S. and Skinner, M. J. (1992). Situational factors and thought processes associated with unprotected sexual intercourse in young gay men. *AIDS, 6*(9), 1021-1030.

Grimley, D. M., DiClemente, C. C., Prochaska, J. O., and Prochaska, G. E. (1995). Preventing adolescent pregnancy, STD and HIV: A promising new approach. *Family Life Educator, 13*(3), 7-15.

Jamner, M. S., Wolitski, R. J., and Corby, N. H. (1997). Impact of a longitudinal community HIV intervention targeting injection drug users' stage of change for condom and bleach use. *American Journal of Health Promotion, 12*(1), 15-24.

Janis, I. L. and Mann, L. (1977). Emergency decision making: A theoretical analysis of responses to disaster warnings. *Journal of Human Stress, 3*(2), 35-45.

Ornstein, M. (1989). Information about AIDS: Sources and responsibility. In M. Ornstein (Ed.), *AIDS in Canada—Knowledge, Behavior, and Attitudes of Adults* (pp. 34-35). Toronto: Institute for Social Research.

Patten, S. and Vollman, A. R. (1999). The social context of HIV risk assumption and risk reduction strategies employed by injection drug users. Masters thesis, University of Calgary.

Prochaska, J. O., DiClemente, C. C., and Norcross, J. C. (1992). In search of how people change: Applications to addictive behaviors. *American Psychologist, 47*(9), 1102-1114.

Prochaska, J. O. and Norcross, J. C. (1994). Comparative conclusions: Toward a transtheoretical therapy. In J. O. Prochaska and J. C. Norcross, *Systems of Psychotherapy: A Transtheoretical Analysis* (pp. 453-493). Pacific Grove: Brooks/ Cole Publishing Company.

Prochaska, J. O. and Velicer, W. F. (1997). The transtheoretical model of health behavior change. *American Journal of Health Promotion, 12*(1), 38-48.

Prochaska, J. O., Velicer, W. F., Rossi, J. S., Goldstein, M., Marcus, B. H., Rakowski, W., Fiore, C., Harlow, L., Redding, C. A., Rosenbloom, D., et al. (1994). Stages of change and decisional balance for 12 problem behaviors. *Health Psychology, 13*(1), 39-46.

Springer, E. (1991). Effective AIDS prevention with active drug users: The harm reduction model. In M. Shernoff (Ed.), *Counseling Chemically Dependent People with HIV Illness* (p. 141). Binghamton, NY: The Haworth Press.

Velicer, W. F., Rossi, J. S., Ruggiero, L., and Prochaska, J. O. (1994). Minimal interventions appropriate for an entire population of smokers. In R. Richmond (Ed.), *Interventions for Smokers: An International Perspective* (pp. 69-92). Baltimore: Williams and Wilkins.

Chapter 4

Utilization of Needle Exchange Programs and Substance Abuse Treatment Services by Injection Drug Users: Social Work Practice Implications of a Harm Reduction Model

Therese Fitzgerald
Timothy Purington
Karen Davis
Faith Ferguson
Lena Lundgren

INTRODUCTION

Working with active injection drug users (IDUs) requires a knowledge of the specific health concerns that should be addressed to optimize the health status of IDUs. Unfortunately, many of these health concerns are not directly addressed by the majority of traditional health care providers. Because of this, it is important for social workers to familiarize themselves with these issues and to be prepared to advocate for users in order to ensure that they receive quality health care. One way of doing this is to employ harm reduction models when working with injection drug users to reduce the health conse-

We gratefully acknowledge the support of the Massachusetts Bureau of Substance Abuse Services and the Robert Wood Johnson Foundation in this research.

Information presented in this chapter was presented at the annual conference of The Society for Social Work Research, January 2002, in a poster presentation titled, "Examination of Service Use by Injection Drug Users in Needle Exchange and Drug Treatment Programs in Massachusetts: 1996-1999."

quences of their injection drug use including HIV infection, hepatitis, overdoses, and abscesses.

The Risk of HIV Infection and Transmission Among Injection Drug Users

Among national AIDS cases, injection drug use is the second most common category of exposure (Prendergast, Urada, and Podus, 2001). One-third of AIDS cases in the United States are caused by injection drug use (Centers for Disease Control, 2002). According to the Centers for Disease Control, infection and transmission of HIV are the result of injection drug users (IDUs) sharing contaminated syringes and drug-injection equipment and through high-risk sexual behaviors (CDC, 2002). Injection drug use is also an important source of HIV transmission to noninjecting persons, as HIV infection can spread from injection drug users to their sexual partners, and from infected mothers to children (Gostin et al., 1997).

When discussing HIV/AIDS services for the drug-using population, one cannot ignore noninjected drugs and alcohol given that alcohol and drugs of all types can impair a person's judgment during the sexual decision-making process (Stein, 1998). However, crack cocaine, cocaine, and heroin use put users at the greatest risk for HIV infection (Stein, 1998). Smoking crack cocaine increases the risk of HIV infection because it is directly related to "increased and prolonged unprotected sexual activity, often in exchange for drugs or money to buy drugs" (Stein, 1998, p. 306). Heroin and cocaine use pose a risk for HIV infection because of the high probability of contracting the virus through shared drug-injection equipment (Stein, 1998). Cocaine use in fact poses an even greater risk of infection than heroin. The high a drug user achieves from cocaine is not as long lasting as the high achieved from heroin resulting in more frequent injection and thus, a higher risk of HIV infection (Stein, 1998).

Although injection drug use is directly related to HIV transmission, it is also associated with other risks and harm, including crime, violence, and the transmission of other diseases such as hepatitis. The following demographic profile of injection drug use and AIDS is based on Massachusetts and national data.

National- and State-Level Data on HIV Infection and Transmission Among IDUs

Although injection drug use has emerged as an important route for HIV transmission, its influence varies by state and region. When compared to the United States, this variability can be seen in the state of Massachusetts, where injection drug use is significantly associated with AIDS cases.

The 2000 Census estimates the national population at 281.5 million, with 69 percent white, 12 percent African Americans, and 12 percent Latinos. Massachusetts, with an overall population of 6.4 million, is 82 percent white, 5 percent African American, and 7 percent Latino. Thus, Massachusetts has a lower percentage of African-American and Latino residents compared to the national percentages (Massachusetts Department of Public Health, 2001a).

Nationwide, IDUs are more likely to be male (75 percent), African American (47 percent), and relatively young (45 percent between ages thirty and thirty-nine). The average age of IDUs in the state of Massachusetts (34.5 years) reflects the national average. The majority of IDUs in Massachusetts are male (68 percent) and white (67 percent), followed by Latino (24 percent), and African American (9 percent) (Massachusetts Department of Public Health, 2001a). IDUs in Massachusetts are also more likely to be high school graduates, not homeless, unemployed, and publicly insured (Lundgren et al., 2001).

Overall, Massachusetts ranks eighth in diagnosed AIDS cases in the United States. From 1992 to 2000, injection drug use was the primary exposure route for the majority of AIDS diagnoses in Massachusetts. In 2000, injection drug use was responsible for 31 percent of AIDS cases in Massachusetts, compared to 20 percent of AIDS cases in the United States. Furthermore, a higher percentage of AIDS cases are reported among IDUs in Massachusetts than the number of cases among IDUs in the United States as a whole (Massachusetts Department of Public Health, 2001a; Massachusetts HIV/AIDS Surveillance Program, 2001).

African-American and Latino IDUs in Massachusetts are disproportionately impacted by HIV and AIDS, with rates that are considerably higher than the rates found among white IDUs. Among those Massachusetts residents living with HIV/AIDS in which injection drug use has been identified as the mode of transmission, 24 percent are African American, and 35 percent are Latino. Approximately 59 percent of all Massachusetts residents living with HIV/AIDS, in which injection drug use was the mode of transmission, are persons of color even though persons of color account for just 12 percent of the general population in the state (Massachusetts Department of Public Health, 2001a).

National- and State-Level Data on IDUs in Drug Treatment

Injection drug use is an important factor in the decision to use substance abuse treatment. In Massachusetts, 27 percent of all admissions to substance abuse treatment programs reported injection drug use in 2000. Among all IDU admissions in 2000, the average age was thirty-four, 71 percent were male, 70 percent were white, 20 percent were Latino, and 7 percent were African American. The majority of these IDUs (89 percent) reported injecting heroin in the past year (Massachusetts Department of Public Health, 2001b; McCarty, LaPrade, and Botticelli, 1996).

The Massachusetts profile of IDUs in drug treatment is consistent with national findings which show that IDUs using drug treatment tend to be male, younger, and report heroin as the primary drug of choice. Due to the importance of these findings, the state of Massachusetts has declared injection drug use as a priority for increased services, treatment, and funding, with special emphasis on targeting the observed racial and ethnic differences (McCarty, LaPrade, and Botticelli, 1996).

THE HARM REDUCTION PHILOSOPHY

Given the current modes of HIV transmission in the United States, most social work case managers working in the field of substance abuse will encounter clients who have contracted HIV through the use of an infected syringe. Though some of these clients may be practicing abstinence, the likelihood is high that many will still be using drugs. Therefore, social work practitioners should be informed of the relevance of the harm reduction model and find ways to incorporate this model into their practice.

Description of the Harm Reduction Philosophy

The term "harm reduction" refers to a nonjudgmental approach to working with injection drug users (Des Jarlais, 1995; Sorge, 1991; Springer, 1991). In this model, HIV is considered a greater danger to individuals and society than substance abuse. Priority is given to reducing the risk of HIV transmission rather than focusing exclusively on abstinence from drugs (Canadian Centre on Substance Abuse National Working Group on Policy, 1996). In harm reduction a drug user is not expected to embrace a goal of abstinence in order to receive services.

No universally accepted definition or prescription for implementing harm reduction exists (Canadian Centre on Substance Abuse National Working Group on Policy, 1996). Because of this, it is important to understand the principles that guide harm reduction programming. The Harm Reduction Coalition (1998) identifies the following set of principles to consider in establishing harm reduction programming:

- Accepts, for better and for worse, that licit and illicit drug use is part of our world and chooses to work to minimize its harmful effects rather than simply ignore or condemn them.
- Understands drug use as a complex, multifaceted phenomenon that encompasses a continuum of behaviors from severe abuse to total abstinence, and acknowledges that some ways of using drugs are clearly safer than others.
- Establishes quality of individual and community life and well-being—not necessarily cessation of all drug use—as the criteria for successful interventions and policies.
- Calls for the nonjudgmental, noncoercive provision of services and resources to people who use drugs and the communities in which they live in order to assist them in reducing attendant harm.
- Ensures that drug users and those with a history of drug use routinely have a real voice in the creation of programs and policies designed to serve them.
- Affirms drugs users themselves as the primary agents of reducing the harms of their drug use, and seeks to empower users to

share information and support one another in strategies which
meet their actual conditions of use.
- Recognizes that the realities of poverty, class, racism, social isolation, past trauma, sex-based discrimination, and other social
  inequalities affect both people's vulnerability to and capacity
  for effectively dealing with drug-related harm.
- Does not attempt to minimize or ignore the real and tragic harm
  and danger associated with licit and illicit drug use.

The Harm Reduction Coalition (1998), based in New York City
and Oakland, California, defines harm reduction as:

> a set of practical strategies that reduce negative consequences of
> drug use, incorporating a spectrum of strategies from safer use,
> to managed use, to abstinence. Harm reduction strategies meet
> drug users "where they're at," addressing conditions of use
> along with the use itself.

In the harm reduction model, substance abuse treatment may be
viewed along a continuum. Rather than forcing a goal of abstinence
on the consumer, the individuals are allowed to choose whether abstinence is a goal for them. Successful treatment for some might involve
avoiding sharing injection equipment or switching from injecting to
oral or smokable drugs (Springer, 1991). For others, decreasing the
amount of drugs consumed is effective substance abuse treatment in
the harm reduction model. Achieving drug-free status is also an important goal in harm reduction when the individual freely chooses it.

Because harm reduction takes a nonjudgmental approach to drug
use, widespread implementation often requires tolerant drug policies.
For this reason, the United States has been slow to widely embrace
harm reduction. Examples of harm reduction strategies that have
been implemented in various countries include: needle exchange,
methadone treatment, education and outreach, and treatment programs that are not solely focused on abstinence (Canadian Centre on
Substance Abuse National Working Group on Policy, 1996).

History of the Harm Reduction Model

The origins of harm reduction are thought to be from Merseyside,
England (Springer, 1991). In the early days of the AIDS epidemic,

policymakers in England recognized the need for a public health response to HIV transmission among IDUs. In 1988, the Advisory Council on the Misuse of Drugs stated: "The spread of HIV is a greater danger to individual and public health than drug misuse. Accordingly, we believe that services which aim to minimize HIV risk behavior by all available means should take precedence in development plans" (as cited in Brettle, 1995). The model developed in the subsequent years became known as the Merseyside Harm Reduction Model (Springer, 1991).

NEEDLE EXCHANGE PROGRAMS

In the United States, the most commonly known harm reduction programs are needle exchange programs (NEPs). A group of intravenous drug users started a needle exchange program in the Netherlands in 1984 in an effort to prevent the spread of hepatitis B (Buning, 1991). In the United States, needle-exchange programs were formed in the late 1980s in Tacoma, Washington, and Boston, Massachusetts, by AIDS activists (Lane, 1993). In 1986, Jon Parker, a former IDU, began exchanging used syringes for new ones in New Haven, Connecticut, and Boston, Massachusetts (Lane, 1993). Two years later, David Purchase began the first needle exchange program in Tacoma that had community involvement (Lane, 1993). In 1998, approximately 131 programs were known to exist in the United States (Singh et al., 2001).

Legal Issues and Governmental Restrictions on Needle Exchange Programs in the United States

As of 1998, thirty-three states had NEPs operating in their communities. The following seven states with NEPs explicitly authorize such programs: California, Connecticut, the District of Columbia, Hawaii, Maryland, New Mexico, and Rhode Island. Although Maine and Vermont did not have any NEPs in 1998, state statutes authorized them. Many other states have made no law expressly prohibiting NEPs, and courts, local programs, or both have interpreted the existing laws as permitting them. Of these, the states with NEPs in 1998 were as follows: Alaska, Arizona, Colorado, Georgia, Illinois, Indiana, Kansas, Louisiana, Massachusetts, Michigan, Minnesota, Montana, New Hampshire, New Jersey, New York, North Carolina, Ohio, Oklahoma, Oregon, Pennsylvania, Tennessee, Texas, Utah, Washington, and Wisconsin, as well as Puerto Rico. The remaining states had no known NEPs in operation in 1998 (Kaiser Family Foundation, 2001).

Current substance abuse treatment approaches stress abstinence from drug use as the primary desired treatment outcome. In terms of HIV prevention and education, Congress has also expressed reluctance to support programs that seemingly promote or encourage drug use (Burris, 1992). Therefore, federal and state policies often use ambiguous language when discussing programs and approaches based on harm reduction. Instead of directly referring to "harm reduction," written materials might use the term "risk reduction." This ambiguity permits different interpretations of what "risk reduction" may mean and thus, places a burden of decision on needle-exchange workers.

In 1997, the Clinton administration supported an official inquiry on the efficacy of needle-exchange programs in reducing HIV transmission and its impact on illegal substance use. Although the final report acknowledged that needle exchange was effective in reducing the risk for HIV transmission, the report did not comment on the role of needle exchange in patterns of drug use. Donna Shalala, then Secretary for the Department of Health and Human Services, concluded that the federal government would continue to restrict funding for nationwide NEPs and further recommended that support and funding for NEPs should remain at the community level (Friedman, 1998).

Despite the government's report demonstrating the effectiveness of harm reduction-based programs on reducing HIV risk, the United States federal government restricts funding and support for national NEPs (Friedman, 1998). This decision is based primarily on the federal government's reluctance to endorse a method that does not encourage abstinence from illegal drugs. The prevailing federal governmental philosophy holds individuals responsible for their own deliberate actions, and therefore primarily supports policies of abstinence or punishment for drug use (Burris, 1992). This limited position of the government is reflected by a persistent refusal to approve a federal policy supporting and funding national NEPs.

Because injection drug use is clearly defined as a violation of existing drug laws, NEPs operating from a harm-reduction perspective are in direct conflict with criminal drug laws (Burris, 1992). Gostin (1998) discussed how these laws operate in direct opposition of each other, producing tension between the criminal justice and substance abuse communities. The federal government currently remains divided between national public health and law enforcement efforts, and as a result, needle-exchange policy typically originates from state public health departments and legislatures (Gostin, 1998; Burris, 1992).

The Controlled Substances Act of Massachusetts (Chapter 94C, Section 27) restricts the sale, exchange, delivery, and possession of hypodermic syringes to persons not lawfully granted access to syringes and requires a physician's prescription to purchase syringes (General Laws of Massachusetts, 2002). The final clause in the Controlled Substances Act establishes the rules and regulations for NEPs in Massachusetts. These state-approved programs exempt individuals legally registered with the exchange from criminal charges resulting from the distribution, possession, and exchange of hypodermic needles. However, the Massachusetts law does recommend that persons participating in needle exchange be referred to substance abuse treatment (General Laws of Massachusetts, 2002).

The National Association of Social Workers (NASW) Position on Harm Reduction and Needle Exchange

The National Association of Social Workers (NASW), founded in 1955, is the largest and most recognized organization of professional social workers in the world representing 150,000 members from the United States and abroad (National Association of Social Workers, 2002). The association seeks to enhance the well-being of individuals, families, and communities while developing, protecting, and promoting the practice of social work and social workers (National Association of Social Workers, 2002).

In *Social Work Speaks,* a compilation of policy statements published by the NASW, social workers are urged to continue their leadership role in combating the negative effects of HIV/AIDS by offering services to at-risk populations including substance users (Mayden and Nieves, 2000). The NASW stresses the importance of reaching out to the most vulnerable populations who often lack access to conventional programs that offer education and prevention services and educating "clients about risk reduction behaviors, including safer sexual practices and harm reduction" (Mayden and Nieves, 2000, p. 5). Specifically, NASW policy states that "needle exchange programs should be part of a comprehensive HIV prevention program for drug users, including efforts to reduce sexual risk behaviors, to increase the quantity and quality of drug abuse treatment, and to reduce drug use in the community" (Mayden and Nieves, 2000, p. 5).

MASSACHUSETTS STATE TREATMENT NEEDS ASSESSMENT PROGRAM

Description of the Project

The findings presented as follows are from the Massachusetts State Treatment Needs Assessment Program (STNAP) titled, "Service Gaps and Substance Abuse Treatment Needs among African-American and White Injection Drug Users: A Longitudinal Study." STNAP is a multiyear needs assessment that examines the gaps in services to African-American and white injection drug users in five domains:

1. health care,
2. health insurance,
3. housing,
4. substance abuse treatment services, and
5. employment.

The following is a presentation of findings from a study of IDUs enrolled in substance abuse treatment services and NEPs in Massachusetts. The findings provide evidence of the value in using harm reduction models when working with injection drug users.

The data presented originate from two databases. The first database includes all IDU admissions to all substance abuse treatment programs licensed by the Massachusetts Department of Public Health, Bureau of Substance Abuse Services (BSAS) for the years 1996 through 1999. This database has been recognized as one of the relatively few statewide drug-treatment databases that is both comprehensive and accurate enough to permit detailed exploration of drug-treatment utilization (McCarty et al., 1998). The second database is from the Massachusetts Department of Public Health, HIV/AIDS Bureau and consists of intake and needle exchange data collected on clients who have used state-licensed NEPs in Massachusetts.

The population using substance abuse treatment includes 36,691 IDUs age eighteen to seventy-five who were admitted to licensed Bureau of Substance Abuse Services treatment programs in Massachusetts between 1996 and 1999 and who reported having ever injected drugs. The population of NEP participants included 4,332 clients of whom 3,377 also entered treatment for substance abuse in a licensed program in Massachusetts between 1996 and 1999.

Table 4.1 provides a breakdown of the demographics for: (1) those who entered needle exchange programs only; (2) those who entered both Massachusetts NEPs and state-licensed substance abuse treatment programs and; (3) those who entered the state-licensed drug treatment programs only. Variables beyond basic demographic information (i.e., race or sex) are limited in the needle exchange database, thus limiting our ability to investigate factors such as employment status, homelessness, and the like for NEP clients who did not enter state-licensed drug treatment programs.

Findings

Needle exchange users were more likely to enter substance abuse treatment than IDUs who did not use needle exchange. Specifically, starting in 1996, 4,332 clients utilized NEPs in Massachusetts. Of those, 78 percent also entered treatment for substance abuse in a licensed program in Massachusetts between 1996 and 1999. Nine percent (9 percent) of the substance abuse treatment clients had also utilized a needle exchange program at some point between 1996 and 1999. IDUs who used both needle exchange and some substance abuse treatment programs utilized NEP over a longer period of time (1.8 years versus 1.6 years for those in NEP alone). In addition, those using both programs had higher rates of exchanging dirty needles per year than IDUs utilizing NEP alone—4.8 versus 3.5.

What were the differences between those IDUs who used drug treatment only, those who used needle exchange only, and those who used both services? Table 4.1 shows that, although age is similar across groups, the groups differ in gender and race.

TABLE 4.1. Demographics

	Needle Exchange Programs (NEPs) only (N = 955)	Both NEP and State- Licensed Drug Treatment Programs (N = 3,377)	State- Licensed Drug Treatment Programs only (N = 33,314)
Race			
White	55%	77%	67%
African American	25%	11%	10%
Latino	20%	12%	23%
Gender			
Male	65%	73%	68%
Female	35%	27%	32%
Age	36.2%	35.7%	35.3%
Education			
Less than high school	Not available	18%	28%
High school graduate	Not available	48%	47%
More than high school	Not available	34%	25%
Homelessness	Not available	40%	31%
Employment (full- or part-time)	Not available	32%	27%
Drug injection			
Injected in the prior month	Not available	85%	73%
Injected in the prior year	Not available	84%	75%

Specifically, of those enrolled in NEPs only (N = 955) 55 percent were white, 25 percent were African American, and 20 percent were Latino. Sixty-five percent of those enrolled in NEPs only were male and 35 percent were female. There were 3,377 people who had used both NEPs and state-licensed substance abuse treatment. Of these, 77 percent were white, 11 percent were African American, and 12 percent were Latino. Seventy-three percent of those using both NEPs and drug treatment were male and 27 percent were female. Of those who were enrolled in state-licensed substance abuse treatment programs only (N = 33,314), 67 percent were white, 10 percent African American, and 23 percent Latino. For the group who entered drug treatment only, 68 percent were male and 32 percent were female.

Those who used both programs had more years of education, on average, compared to those who only used state-licensed substance abuse treatment. Also, those who used both programs were more likely to have ever been employed, to have ever been homeless, and to have recently injected drugs.

Needle Exchange Program Use Is Associated with Higher Levels of Substance Abuse Treatment Entry

Drug treatment is a vital method of HIV prevention, not only because it results in a decrease in drug-using behaviors, but also because it offers a way to educate and counsel clients who are at the greatest risk for HIV (Stein, 1998). However, social work case managers may be discouraged rather than encouraged by what many view as a "revolving door" phenomenon in which clients continue to cycle in and out of drug treatment.

Addiction is a chronic disease where one treatment may not be sufficient for recovery. "Because of the chronic, relapsing nature of addiction, multiple treatment episodes can better be understood in terms of cyclic process of recovery rather than as failed efforts" (Hser et al., 1997). According to Hser et al. (1997), "cumulative treatment participation" may be required in order for a change in drug use to take effect over time. For many drug users, repeated treatment episodes may be necessary over the long-term in order to effectively diminish drug use (Hser et al., 1997).

Our study of the Massachusetts substance abuse treatment and NEP data shows that utilization of needle exchange by IDUs may enhance this "cumulative treatment participation." The findings demonstrate that IDUs who utilized both NEPs and state-licensed drug treatment programs had, on average, more substance abuse treatment admissions than IDUs using state-licensed substance abuse treatment alone. Those using NEPs in addition to state-licensed drug treatment had an average of 4.3 drug treatment admissions compared to 3.2 drug treatment admissions for those who only entered drug treatment.

Needle Exchange Use Is Associated with Utilization of Higher-Quality Drug Treatment Services

When compared with detoxification only, entry into *any* form of drug abuse treatment (e.g., long-term residential, drug-free outpatient, methadone maintenance) is associated with more positive outcomes (Gerstein and Harwood, 1990; Hien and Scheier, 1996; Simpson and Sells, 1990). Our findings establish a link between NEP participation and entry into higher-quality drug treatment. The data presented in Table 4.2 indicate that clients who used both needle exchange and drug treatment services were more likely to enter methadone maintenance, residential, and outpatient counseling drug treatment than those who did not use needle exchange. In addition, those who only entered drug treatment and did not use needle exchange services were more likely to enter the less-effective drug treatment trajectory of using detoxification only without any follow-up drug treatment.

Specifically, those who utilized NEPs in addition to drug treatment were more likely to enter: methadone maintenance (33 percent compared to 26 percent for those in drug treatment only); residential drug treatment (23 percent compared to 20 percent for those in drug treatment only) and; outpatient counseling (41 percent compared to 35 percent for those in drug treatment only). Those who did not use needle exchange were more likely to enter the less effective drug treat-

TABLE 4.2. Substance Abuse Treatment Utilization

Substance Abuse Treatment Modality	Both NEP and State-Licensed Drug Treatment Programs (N = 3,377)		State-Licensed Drug Treatment Programs Only (N = 33,314)	
	N	%	N	%
Detoxification Only *	1,026	30	12,433	37
Detoxification *	2,585	77	23,716	71
Methadone Maintenance *	1,103	33	8,651	26
Residential *	780	23	6,624	20
Outpatient Counseling *	1,382	41	11,800	35

Mean number of admissions (Standard deviation) *
* p < .001

ment trajectory of detoxification only (37 percent compared to 30 percent for those using both NEPs and drug treatment).

To summarize, those who did not use NEPs were more likely to have been in detoxification treatment only, and less likely to use other treatment modalities that are known to be more effective. Thus, Massachusetts IDUs who were exposed to harm reduction services in the form of NEPs accessed more effective drug treatment modalities than those who did not receive NEP services.

These findings underscore the importance of the harm reduction model in improving entry into drug treatment. Not only are those using NEP services entering treatment more frequently, they are also entering more effective treatment modalities than those individuals who have not been exposed to NEP services.

PRACTICE IMPLICATIONS

Harm reduction is a philosophy that informs practice. Social work case managers have a unique opportunity to engage in a harm reduction dialogue with IDUs to reduce the negative consequences of drug use in ways that have not been undertaken by other health-care professionals. Health care providers may fear that talking about overdosing or using clean needles will cause a person to relapse or will be construed as promoting drug use. Therefore, IDUs may not get the medically necessary information they need in a traditional drug treatment setting.

Strategies such as multiple contacts and sustained relationships allow the social worker to build credibility as a provider and to respond to the more immediate health concerns of the IDU. Therefore, if the IDU's immediate health threat is fear of overdosing or access to clean needles, it is important to meet the client "where he or she is at," a central concept in the social work philosophy, which can lead to more lasting harm reduction strategies over the long-term.

Social work practitioners need to be aware that a pattern of use and reuse of substance abuse treatment modalities by IDUs is an acceptable treatment path for clients in their efforts to reduce or stop their drug use. Although possibly frustrating for the practitioner, multiple substance abuse treatment entries are often necessary given the chronic nature of addiction. The findings from the study of IDUs in

Massachusetts indicate that "cumulative treatment participation" (Hser et al., 1997) is enhanced by the harm reduction model in the form of needle exchange programs.

IDUs often experience discrimination and harassment in many parts of their lives. As a result of their current or past drug use, many IDUs experience coercive health care providers, have lost the right to vote, have had their children removed from their homes, are unable to secure adequate housing, or are viewed by society in a dehumanizing manner. Because of these experiences, many IDUs are reluctant to disclose, even to the most well-intentioned helper, their current drug use. By incorporating a harm reduction strategy, social work practitioners will be better able to treat the chronic nature of the clients' addictions as well as assist them in accessing more effective treatment modalities.

Our study demonstrates that clients who have utilized needle exchange services were more likely to have accessed more effective drug treatment modalities, such as methadone maintenance and residential treatment, than those clients not enrolled in NEPs. The implication is that harm reduction strategies are instrumental in bridging the way to higher-quality drug treatment.

Limitations of the Harm Reduction Model in Practice

Some social work case managers may have difficulty incorporating harm reduction strategies into their practice because the model does not require abstinence from drugs and alcohol on the part of the client. Many traditional treatment programs require a client's abstinence before allowing participation in the program. However, those clients who are able to maintain sobriety throughout treatment often suffer from one or more relapses. Given the chronic, relapsing nature of drug addiction, social work practitioners can use harm reduction as a means of reducing the risk of HIV transmission by helping clients reduce the harmful effects of their drug use and promoting healthy behaviors among active users (Stein, 1998). Social workers can also use the model to understand "revolving door" clients who are trying to reduce the harmful effects of drug use.

One cannot ignore the legal and governmental restrictions that have been placed on NEPs in this country. Many social workers practice in states where NEPs are illegal or where funding for harm reduction services is limited. However, social workers have an obligation to become leaders in lobbying the appropriate state, local, and federal levels of government on behalf of people with HIV/AIDS to improve the quality of lives, protect their civil liberties, and to increase funding for HIV/AIDS services and research (Mayden and Nieves, 2000).

Although harm reduction strategies may meet with opposition for a variety of reasons in the agencies and towns in which social workers are practicing, according to the NASW, "social workers must address community norms that create barriers to disseminating accurate information" (Mayden and Nieves, 2000, p. 6). Given the important role that harm reduction program services, specifically NEPs, play in providing necessary services to at-risk populations, social workers need to be actively engaged in efforts to ensure that these types of services are accessible to their clients.

CONCLUSION

Social work case managers have a unique opportunity when working with vulnerable populations such as injection drug users to serve as a liaison to the health care community and to provide information that is not routinely covered by traditional medical providers. By remaining neutral with the information provided, social work case managers can send a strong message to injection drug users that their health care needs are understood and that they are accepted "where they are at" in the recovery process.

Given the coercive relationships many IDUs experience in dealing with health care providers, the law, and other government agencies such as child protective services agencies, IDUs have built up mistrust of many professionals they need to access for help. By working from a harm reduction model, a practitioner can work on improving the health of IDUs while at the same time building trust with the goal of assisting them in their efforts to reduce their drug use and risky behaviors over the long-term, important goals in curbing the transmission of HIV infection among injection drug users.

Also, given that biases and attitudes of the social worker can get in the way of effective substance abuse treatment (Stein, 1998), social workers need to address their own feelings toward active drug users. As the policy position of the NASW emphasizes, it is important that social workers find a way to reach out to "vulnerable populations—those not reached by traditional prevention and education programs" (Mayden and Nieves, 2000, p. 5). Active IDUs certainly fall into the realm of a vulnerable population and harm reduction program services offer a unique way of working with this population in ways that abstinence-based programs cannot.

In addition, it is important for social work case managers not only to screen and counsel clients for risky behaviors around their drug use but also for their risky sexual behaviors (Stein, 1998). In fact, more research needs to be conducted in this area to determine whether drug-use harm reduction also leads to harm reduction in other behaviors such as risky sexual behavior. Finally, our study indicates a further need to explore racial and gender differences in drug treatment and NEP utilization patterns.

REFERENCES

Brettle, R. P. (1995). Harm reduction for IDU-related HIV. In Brettle, R. P. *Human immunodeficiency virus: The Edinburgh epidemic* [electronic version]. Retrieved March 6, 2002, from <http://www/link.med.ac.uk/RIDU/Hxharm.htm>.

Buning, E. C. (1991). Effects of Amsterdam needle and syringe exchange. *International Journal of the Addictions, 26*(12), 1303-1311.

Burris, S. (1992). HIV education and the law: A critical review. *Law, Medicine, and Health Care, 20*(4), 377-391.

Canadian Centre on Substance Abuse National Working Group on Policy (1996). Harm reduction: Concepts and practice, A policy discussion paper. Retrieved March 7, 2002, from <http://www.ccsa.ca/docs/wgharm.htm>.

Centers for Disease Control (1998). Update: Syringe exchange programs. United States, 1997. *Morbidity and Mortality Weekly Report, 47*(31), August 14, 652-655.

Centers for Disease Control (2002). IDU/HIV prevention: Access to sterile syringes. National Center for HIV, STD and TB Prevention, Divisions of HIV/AIDS Prevention. Retrieved from <http://www.cdc.gov/idu/facts/aed_idu_ acc.htm>.

Des Jarlais, D. C. (1995). Harm reduction: A framework for incorporating science into drug policy. *American Journal of Public Health, 85*, 10-12.

Friedman, D. (1998). A split decision over needle exchanges. *U.S. News and World Report*, May 4, p. 5.

General Laws of Massachusetts (2002). *Controlled Substances Act: Instruments for administering controlled substances by injection*. M.G.L.—Chapter 94C, Section 27. Retrieved January 31, 2002, from <http://www.state.ma.us/legis/laws/mgl/gl-94C-toc.htm>.

Gerstein, D. R., Harwood, H. J., and the Institute of Medicine Committee for Substance Abuse Coverage Study (1990). *Treating drug problems.* Washington, DC: National Academy Press.

Gostin, L.O. (1998). The legal environment impeding access to sterile syringes and needles: The conflict between law enforcement and public health. *Journal of Immune Deficiency Syndrome and Human Retrovirology, 18*(1), 60-70.

Gostin, L. O, Lazzarini, Z., Jones, T. S., and Flaherty, K. (1997). Prevention of HIV/ AIDS and other blood-borne diseases among injection drug users: A national survey on the regulation of syringes and needles. *The Journal of the American Medical Association, 277,* 53-62.

Harm Reduction Coalition (1998). Principles of harm reduction. Retrieved March 8, 2002, from <http://www.harmreduction.org/prince.html>.

Hien, D. and Scheier, J. (1996). Trauma and short-term outcome for women in detoxification. *Journal of Substance Abuse Treatment, 13,* 227-231.

Hser, Y., Anglin, M. D., Grella, C., Longshore, D., and Prendergast, M. L. (1997). Drug treatment careers: A conceptual framework and existing research findings. *Journal of Substance Abuse Treatment, 14*(6), 543-558.

Kaiser Family Foundation (2001). State health facts online, 50 state comparisons: Sterile syring exchange programs, 1998. Retrieved from <www.statehealthfacts. kff.org>.

Lane, S. D., (1993). Needle exchange: A brief history. Retrieved March 8, 2002, from <http://www.aegis.com/law/journals/1993/HKFNE009.html>.

Lundgren, L., Amodeo, M., Ferguson, F., and Davis, K. (2001). Racial and ethnic differences in drug treatment entry of injection drug users in Massachusetts. *Journal of Substance Abuse Treatment, 21*(3), 145-153.

Massachusetts Department of Public Health (2001a). *HIV/AIDS in Massachusetts: An epidemiologic profile, fiscal year 2001.* Boston, MA: HIV/AIDS Bureau, Massachusetts Department of Public Health. Retrieved from <http://www.state. ma.us/dph/aids/research/profile2001/eppro2001.htm>.

Massachusetts Department of Public Health (2001b). *Injection drug use (IDU) in substance abuse treatment.* Boston, MA: Bureau of Substance Abuse Services, Massachusetts Department of Public Health. Retrieved from <http://www.state. ma.us/dph/bsas/documents/fact_sheets/webidu_mar01.pdf>.

Massachusetts HIV/AIDS Surveillance Program (2001). *Massachusetts and U.S. AIDS surveillance statistics: Annual report, 2001.* Boston, MA: Massachusetts HIV/AIDS Surveillance Program, Massachusetts Department of Public Health. Retrieved from <http://www.state.ma.us/dph/cdc/aids/quarterly/mavsus.pdf>.

Mayden, R. and Nieves, R. (2000). *Social work speaks: National association of social workers policy statements, 2000-2003* (Fifth edition). Washington, DC: NASW Press.

McCarty, D., LaPrade, J., and Botticelli, M. (1996). Substance abuse treatment and HIV services: Massachusetts' policies and programs. *Journal of Substance Abuse Treatment, 13*(5), 429-438.

McCarty, D., McGuire, T. G., Harwood, H. J., and Field, T. (1998). Using state information systems for drug abuse services research. *American Behavioral Scientist, 41*(8), 1090-1106.

National Association of Social Workers (2002). The power of social work. National Association of Social Workers Press. Retrieved from <http://www. socialworkers. org/nasw/nasw.pdf>.

Prendergast, M. L., Urada, D., and Podus, D. (2001). Meta-analysis of HIV risk-reduction interventions with drug abuse treatment populations. *Journal of Consulting and Clinical Psychology, 69*(3), 389-405.

Simpson, D. D. and Sells, S. B. (1990). *Opiod addiction and treatment: A 12-year follow up.* Malabar: Krieger Publishing.

Singh, M. P., McKnight, C. A., Paone, D., Titus, S., Des Jarlais, D. C., Krim, M., Purchase, D., Rustard, J., and Solberg, A. (2001). Syringe exchange programs, United States, 1998. *Morbidity and Mortality Weekly Report, 50*(19), 384-387.

Sorge, R. (1991). Harm reduction: A new approach to drug services. *Health/PAC Bulletin* (Asian and Pacific Islander Caucus of Act Up and the Harm Reduction Institute) Winter 1991, 70-75.

Springer, E. (1991). Effective AIDS prevention with active drug users: The harm reduction model. *Journal of Chemical Dependency Treatment, 4*(2), 141-157.

Stein, J. B. (1998). Addressing HIV risks with clients who use drugs. In D. M. Aronstein and B. J. Thompson (Eds.), *HIV and social work: A practitioner's guide* (pp. 303-313). Binghamton, NY: The Haworth Press.

Chapter 5

HIV Prevention Models with Mexican Migrant Farmworkers

Kurt C. Organista

INTRODUCTION

The purpose of this chapter is to discuss HIV prevention and AIDS treatment in Mexican farmworkers in the United States. This unique group of Latinos is generally characterized by extreme poverty, marginalization, exploitation, and vulnerability to a wide variety of economic, health, and social problems. Although they supply essential labor to the lucrative agricultural sector of the U.S. economy, they unfairly toil and struggle with a health-compromising labor system that American workers would not tolerate. The emerging problem of HIV/AIDS in Mexican migrant laborers is embedded within their larger health crisis and must be addressed from a perspective that considers the social, political, and cultural ecology of risk. This chapter reviews pertinent literature, presents a conceptual model of HIV risk, and reviews and suggests viable intervention directions at several ecological levels.

The author would like to acknowledge the invaluable assistance of the following dedicated staff of Salud Para La Gente, Inc., Watsonville, California, for arranging farmworker interviews referred to in this study: Arcadio Viveros, executive director, Maria de Jesus Heredia, health educator and director of HIV prevention program (SalvaSIDA), Guillermina Porraz, community health outreach worker, and Raul Bonilla, health educator.

HIV/AIDS, MEXICAN FARMWORKERS, AND AGRICULTURAL LABOR IN THE UNITED STATES

Sociodemographic Profile

The sociodemographic profile of U.S. farmworkers is estimated at between 2.7 and 4 million in the United States (U.S. Department of Labor, 1990). Although the high population figure included an estimate of family members, the recent trend indicates unaccompanied men and fewer families, in part because growers refuse to house families. As can be seen in the following list from the U.S. Department of Labor (1990, 1998), the annual National Agricultural Worker's Survey (NAWS) has repeatedly documented a migrant labor force that is predominantly Mexican, male, foreign born, non-English speaking, poverty stricken, of very low educational background, and with a high percentage of undocumented workers (Mines, Gabbard, and Steirman, 1997):

Population estimates	2.7 to 4 million
Foreign born	70 percent
Race/ethnic background	
Mexican	65 percent
Other Latino	13 percent
White	18 percent
African American	2 percent
Other	2 percent
Gender (male)	80 percent
Undocumented	52 percent
Education	4 to 7 years
Income (<$10,000 annually)	75 percent
Poverty	60 percent
Illiteracy estimate	10 percent

Such background characteristics interact with a health-compromising labor system to create numerous risk factors and challenges to HIV/ AIDS services and to health care in general for migrant laborers.

The Migrant Farmworker Health Crisis

Death and Injury

The problem of HIV/AIDS in migrant laborers is embedded within the overall health care crisis that has historically plagued farmworkers. For example, in 1987, agricultural labor surpassed mining as the nation's most hazardous occupation with 1,700 deaths (Rust, 1990). According to Schenker (1996), work-related fatalities from agricultural labor are four times higher than in all other American industries combined. Further, work-related deaths and injuries have not declined during the past fifty years as they have for all other American industries such as construction and mining. In California alone an estimated 20,000 disabling injuries occur each year, yet two-thirds of farmers surveyed believe that farmwork is less dangerous than other occupations (Schenker, 1996).

As can be seen in the following list, the pattern of occupational injuries and illnesses affecting farmworkers includes numerous work-related sprains, strains, and accidents; illnesses from acute and chronic pesticide exposure; and several related chronic and infectious diseases ranging from tuberculosis and diabetes to STDs including HIV/AIDS (Napolitano and Goldberg, 1998):

- Work-related injuries/deaths
  musculoskeletal strains and sprains (e.g., back pain)
  falls from ladders
  machine-related accidents (lacerations, amputations, crush injuries)
  electrocution
- Pesticide exposures (acute and chronic) and related illness
  dermatitis
  respiratory problems
  eye problems
  cancer (e.g., brain tumors, lymphoma)
  birth defects (e.g., limb reduction)
- Chronic and infectious diseases
  diabetes
  obesity
  hypertension

tuberculosis
alcoholism (men)
STDs including HIV/AIDS
• Lack of field sanitation
31 percent without toilet and water (Napolitano and Goldberg, 1998; Rust, 1990; Slesinger, 1992)

In fact, researchers at the California Institute for Rural Studies recently published landmark studies on farmworker health including the first-ever statewide survey to include a comprehensive physical examination (Villarejo et al., 2000), as well as a binational health survey of agricultural workers in Mexico and the United States (Mines, Mullenax, and Saca, 2001). In the former survey, it was found that risks for chronic diseases, such as heart disease, stroke, asthma, and diabetes, were very high for a group composed mostly of young Mexican men who would normally be in peak physical condition. It was also found that nearly 70 percent of the 971 participants lacked health insurance, and that only 7 percent were covered by government-funded programs for the poor. Similar findings are reported in the latter survey with the addition that farmworkers receive few, intermittent, and uncoordinated services on *both sides of the border,* limiting opportunities for health promotion and disease prevention.

Despite extremely negative economic and health profiles, farmworker utilization of badly needed health and social services is estimated as low as 4 percent for disability insurance (Social Security), 20 percent for unemployment insurance, and 15 percent for Medicaid, food stamps, and WIC (Mines, Gabbard, and Steirman, 1997). These rates of underutilization are due to a staggering array of structural, cultural, and legal barriers of which service providers and researchers need to be more aware as they approach disease prevention and health promotion with farmworkers.

Lack of Protection Under Federal and State Law

Farmworkers are generally excluded from major federal and state laws designed to protect the health, safety, and economic well-being of American workers (Moses, 1993). For example, the National Labor Relations Act of 1935, which was enacted to guarantee American workers the right to collective bargaining and to form unions, explicitly excludes agricultural laborers. Only in California have farmworkers won the right to unionize.

According to Sakala (1987), the Fair Labor Standards Act of 1938 has legitimized farmworker poverty and facilitated the entrance of farmworker children into the migrant labor system. This act, which regulates minimum wage, time-and-a-half pay for overtime, and child labor, has never been equally applied to farmworkers. As a result, farmworkers are paid below minimum wage, denied overtime wages, and an estimated 100,000 children perform farm labor at younger ages than their American counterparts (Slesinger, 1992). For example, the minimum age at which American children can work nonhazardous jobs is fourteen to sixteen years, yet twelve-year-old Mexican children are permitted to perform hazardous farm labor, outside of school hours, with parental consent (Moses, 1993). Such differential applications of the law undoubtedly contribute to the estimated 300 deaths annually of children and adolescents due to farm injuries (Schenker, 1996).

At the state level, labor contractors, who provide work crews to growers, are recognized as the legal employers of farmworkers. This arrangement dismisses growers from normal employer-related responsibilities to workers and also leaves them at the mercy of frequently unscrupulous contractors that overcharge farmworkers for inadequate housing and dangerous transportation, and frequently cheat them out of wages (e.g., withholding for benefits never delivered; absconding with pay, etc.) (Moses, 1993).

State laws also do not protect farmworkers from the consequences of their hazardous work, chronic underemployment, and frequent unemployment. For example, in twenty-four states, farmworkers are ineligible for workers' compensation insurance when they become injured on the job (Moses, 1993). Six states provide workers' compensation on an optional basis, twelve states provide workers' compensation for the minority of farmworkers that work year-round at the same location, and only eight states provide full coverage. Similarly, the Federal Unemployment Tax Act, which provides income to workers during periods of unemployment, excludes migrant farmworkers (Napolitano and Goldberg, 1998).

Even the Occupational Safety and Health Act of 1970, which regulates health and safety work standards, excludes farmworkers (Moses, 1993). This has resulted in drastic disparities in federal spending on farmworker health and safety. For example, in 1985, the federal government spent $185 per miner as compared to just 30 cents per agricultural worker (Schenker, 1996). Furthermore, a 1982 study by the U.S. Department of Labor found that only 1 percent of OSHA inspections were performed in agricultural settings (Sakala, 1987).

With regard to the major health problem of pesticide exposure, Moses (1993) maintains that the Environmental Protection Agency (EPA) functions more as a pesticide industry collaborator than as a regulator and protector of human health and the environment for a variety of reasons. Although the EPA has issued standards of pesticide protection for farmworkers, there is no formal regulation of standards nor mechanisms for reporting violations (Slesinger, 1992) despite the fact that the EPA estimates 300,000 acute pesticide exposures annually in farm labor (Napolitano and Goldberg, 1998). Pesticide laws are under the control of House and Senate agricultural committees, rather than environmental, health, and labor committees, thus creating a conflict of interest that pits profits against human health and the environment (Moses, 1993). Undoubtedly, the increasingly high proportion of undocumented farmworkers further contributes to the pervasive lack of labor and safety regulation.

Federal Assistance versus Labor Regulation

Rather than attempting to regulate farm labor, Congress has instead chosen to address farmworker problems by developing a number of federally funded assistance programs. Over the past forty years, a continuously expanding budget has been spent on continuously expanding services for a continuously expanding definition of farmworkers. The "big four" programs include Migrant Health, Migrant Education, Migrant Head Start, and a migrant job training program. Unfortunately, these programs are operated by different branches of the government such as the Departments of Health, Education, and Labor, and a general lack of coordination results in numerous gaps and duplications in farmworkers services (Martin and Martin, 1994).

Government assistance programs simply cannot begin to compensate for the lack of farmworker protection under existing laws. A significant part of the problem is that these programs were never designed to ameliorate farmworker problems. Instead they were designed as short-term strategies to assist farmworkers until they were to be displaced by mechanization somewhere in the 1970s (Martin and Martin, 1994). Displacement never happened of course and farmworker needs continue unabated despite occasional federal attention to the problem.

For example, in 1962, the Migrant Health Act was passed to improve health care access for migrant laborers by creating a national network of federally funded clinics. Today, about 400 such clinics exist but reach less than 20 percent of migrant laborers (NACMH, 1995). In addition to the scarcity of such clinics, other barriers include farm labor work schedules, lack of sick leave and transportation, frequent geographical mobility, scarce bilingual services, and high rates of ineligibility due to lack of documentation and policies insensitive to migratory labor. For example, Medicaid eligibility cannot be transferred between states for the few that qualify. The result is sparse and underutilized health resources despite serious farmworker health problems which now include HIV/AIDS.

HIV Risk Profile

Worldwide, migratory labor systems play central roles in the geographical spread of HIV due to migration-related factors such as male migrants being away from home for long periods of time, family breakdown, and increased number of sexual partners, including prostitutes and other men (Hulewicz, 1994). The current HIV/AIDS crisis affecting the African continent is a startling example of how migratory labor, poverty, social and political change interact to create worst-case scenarios (e.g., Decosas et al., 1995; Jochelson, Mothibeli, and Leger, 1994).

Despite the connection between migratory labor and HIV, screenings with migrant laborers in the United States are rare and sporadic. However, the few screenings that have been conducted indicate an epidemic in progress for black farmworkers in the Southeastern states and the making of such an epidemic in Mexican farmworkers. For example, HIV testing in labor camps in Florida and the Carolinas revealed infection rates ranging from 3.5 to an alarming 13 percent in black farmworkers from both the United States and the Caribbean (Organista and Balls Organista, 1997).

Although the results of three HIV screenings with Mexican farm-workers have only found infection rates between 0 and less than 2 percent (CDC, 1988; López and Ruiz, 1995; Carrier and Magaña, 1991), these studies also documented the presence of significant precursors to an AIDS epidemic in this population. In López and Ruiz's (1995) HIV screening of 176 Mexican farmworkers in Northern California, they found a 9 percent history of STDs, two active cases of syphilis, and noted that 9 percent of female respondents reported having sex with a partner using injection drugs. Also, in their screening of 2,000 migrant laborers, Carrier and Magaña (1991) noted that epidemics of syphilis and chancroid had recently occurred in migrant laborers and prostitutes in the Orange County area of Southern California. For example, between 1981 and 1983, 271 cases of chancroid were seen at the county STD clinic where Carrier and Magaña conducted their investigation, as compared to zero cases of chancroid in the previous year (Blackmore et al., 1985). Migrant men accounted for 266 of the 271 cases of chancroid with female prostitutes comprising the remaining five cases.

One screening of 151 drug using farmworkers in the Delmarva Peninsula of Delaware found a prevalence rate of 4 percent or six farmworkers with HIV (Inciardi et al., 1999). Of these six, four were Mexican who each had a history of trading sex for money or drugs. Hence, multiple risk factors need to be considered.

RESEARCH-INFORMED UNDERSTANDING OF HIV RISK

The following review of HIV risk factors in Mexican migrant laborers is based on a review of the literature (Organista and Balls Organista, 1997) and previous empirical surveys and qualitative research. It was the goal of this research to blend both quantitative and qualitative methods in a mutually informative, interactive fashion.

Quantitative Survey Research

Organista and associates conducted a pilot survey of eighty-seven Mexican migrant laborers (Organista et al., 1996) in preparation for a five-site, statewide survey of 501 migrant laborers that was carried out in 1994 (Organista et al., 1997a). Both surveys were conducted in small, remote "sending communities" in Jalisco, Mexico, with historically high rates of out-migration to the United States. Participants were adult migrants who have lived and worked in the United States during the major years of the AIDS epidemic. These migrants worked in a variety of capacities including farmwork and urban-based day labor and unskilled service-sector jobs. The descriptive goal of the research was to assess HIV/AIDS-related knowledge, attitudes, beliefs, and behaviors, and the analytic component was to explore predictors of condom use.

Qualitative Research

Twenty-one semistructured, private, qualitative interviews were conducted with adult male farmworkers in Northern California, as well as two outreach workers serving these men. Two open-ended meetings with HIV prevention program staff serving the farmworkers were also conducted. In addition, a focus group with outreach workers providing HIV prevention education to urban-based Mexican migrant day laborers was also conducted.

These qualitative data were collected to make better sense of the risk factors documented in the survey research and literature.

HIV RISK FACTORS IN MEXICAN MIGRANT LABORERS

Prostitution Use

Organista et al. (1997a) found that 44 percent of 342 male respondents reported sex with prostitutes while working in the United States. Interestingly, married men in the survey were as likely as single men to use prostitutes but less likely to use condoms, underscoring significant risk to wives. Results of qualitative interviews conveyed that *mujeres de la calle* (women of the street) are readily available, inexpensive, and used as sexual outlets sporadically and regularly:

> Women who sell their bodies, I use them every fifteen days or so. Or if I have enough money, right? Fifteen, twenty dollars; it's not expensive. There are plenty available. All you have to do is go to the bars or where one knows. For example, there are many homes, let's say, where one can find the women.

Well, I have experienced many women and have gotten diseases four times. Not AIDS but venereal diseases.

With regard to the complex ways that culture and migratory labor influence behavior, it was also found that 13 percent of the men surveyed reported participating in a male bonding ritual in which several migrant men have sex with the same prostitute in succession. After such an experience, these men refer to themselves as *hermanos de leche* (milk brothers), presumably for sharing sperm. This ritual was also documented by Magaña (1991) who interviewed fifty male Mexican migrants and thirty-eight injection drug-using female prostitutes. Magaña reported that the prostitutes actively solicited the men at the labor camps, bars, and other locations where they congregated, especially on payday. Efforts to promote condom use with prostitutes will need to consider the complex ways that migratory labor and Mexican culture frame this especially salient HIV exposure category.

Sex Between Men

Surveys of Mexican migrants inquiring about sex between men report rates ranging from only 2 to 3.5 percent (Lafferty, 1991; López and Ruiz, 1995; Organista et al., 1997a). Although these survey interviews were private and conducted by male interviewers, the figures most likely underestimate this taboo behavior. For example, when presurvey focus groups were conducted with migrant men to discuss the topic, all participants acknowledged the occasional practice of heterosexual *macho* men occasionally having sex with other men when women are unavailable. But when asked directly about such personal experience, all denied it.

Carrier (1995) has written extensively about the construction of (homo)sexuality in Mexico versus the United States in ways that are informative to HIV prevention research and services. Consistent with the focus groups, Carrier has long noted that masculine Mexican men that occasionally play the active inserter role with passive, effeminate men may continue to self-identify as heterosexual and lead such public lives. Such culture-based sexual behaviors are bound to be influenced by the experience of migratory labor in which sex between men probably increases. For example, Bronfman and Minello (1992) conducted in-depth, qualitative interviews with Mexican migrants and concluded that homosexual contact increases with migration due to factors such as extended periods of loneliness, isolation, emotional deprivation, and greater sexual freedom in the United States.

Qualitative interviews with heterosexual-identified farmworkers corroborate the practice of sex between men, short of admitting any such personal experience, and convey that certain men become known and pursued for sex.

> There was a *maricon* [pejorative term for homosexual] where I worked and he pursued the men in the fields and they kissed him like a woman. And there was another man who liked him and we would find them hugging and kissing and one time having sex in a car as if they were a man and a woman. They used to give this guy money, they bought him clothes, his lunch, they would invite him to the lunch truck. He was homosexual but the others had wives.

Interviews with gay-identified farmworkers conveyed the same information but with the addition of personal experience.

> I was eighteen when I came to the United States and I already knew that I was gay. Everybody around me also knew because I was *obvio* [slang term for effeminate literally meaning "obvious"]. Well, anyways, everyday men would joke with me about having sex but they were really serious. In just a few weeks I was having a lot of sex with different men.

Alcohol and Substance Abuse

The connection between substance use and HIV risk has been well documented in the HIV/AIDS literature although little information is available on migrant laborers. This is unfortunate given that migratory labor appears to place workers at high risk for alcohol and drug abuse/dependence. For example, in the only epidemiological study to assess psychiatric disorders in farmworkers, Alderete et al. (2000) found that among the 500 men assessed, 9 percent had a lifetime prevalence rate of alcohol dependence, and 12 percent had a lifetime prevalence of any substance abuse/dependence disorder. The following interview excerpts convey the frequent problem of alcohol and substance use in Mexican male farmworkers.

Yes, here [in the United States] one can become ruined because I had a good job with this gringo in Santa Cruz, right? I was doing well, they paid me eighty dollars a day and in a few months I had my own car. But then I got together with some friends to drink, right? "Hey, let's go drink us some beers! Let's go to the bar." Well, the police saw me leave the bar drunk and get into my car and they stopped me without a license or anything and I lost my car and my job too.

About three years ago I tried it two times [heroin] but it didn't have any effect on me. I didn't feel good with that. On the contrary, I felt sick in the stomach and right after I wanted to vomit all day and I lasted that way with sore bones. Who needs that?

With regard to HIV risk and substance use, McBride et al. (1999) conducted a study to examine the health beliefs model (HBM) (Rosenstock, Strecher, and Becker, 1988) in a sample of 846 drug-using migrant farmworkers, and their sex partners, in the Delmarva Peninsula of Delaware. During the past six months, 98 percent of the study sample had used crack cocaine and 2 percent had injected drugs. Mexican farmworkers comprised about 50 percent of the sample, blacks 40 percent, and whites 10 percent. The HBM was partially tested by assessing the relation between perceived susceptibility to contracting HIV and various risk and protective behaviors.

Results revealed that 78 percent of the sample perceived only a less than 25 percent chance of contracting HIV, and that Mexicans had the lowest perceptions of risk as compared to their black and white counterparts. McBride and colleagues did find partial support for the HBM in that those migrants with the highest perceived susceptibility also had the highest rates of safer sex and condom use. For example, only 8 percent of those perceiving no risk practiced safer sex versus 18 percent of those perceiving a greater than 75 percent chance of contracting HIV. Thus, the need to increase perceptions of risk in general, but especially for Mexican migrant laborers, is warranted.

Needle Sharing

Sharing needles is an interesting risk factor for Mexican migrants because economic and cultural factors combine to result in the occasional practice of lay "therapeutic injections" of vitamins and antibiotics. In Mexico, it is legal and common for people to purchase and use hypodermic needles to medicate themselves and family members. This practice continues in the United States, especially given the low access to affordable health care.

For example, Lafferty (1991) found that 20 percent of 411 Mexican farmworkers reported receiving lay therapeutic injections. Of these, 3.5 percent reported sharing the needle with family members. In contrast, only 2.9 percent of the sample reported illegal injection drug use. More recently, McVea (1997) found that 12 percent of 532 Mexican farmworkers surveyed admitted to lay injection with antibiotics or vitamins. Thus, HIV prevention messages aimed at needle sharing must not be confined to illegal drug use.

Gender and HIV Risk

As mentioned earlier, the wives and girlfriends of migrant men are at risk for HIV due to the risky behaviors of their male sex partners. Unfortunately, risk for these women is exacerbated by their very low knowledge of STDs (Schoonover Smith, 1988) and cultural prohibitions to HIV prevention strategies such as condom use. For example, Organista et al. (1997a) found that migrants in general and female migrants in particular believed that women would be seen as promiscuous for carrying condoms. As a result, 75 percent of the 159 women surveyed reported "never" carrying condoms as compared to 41.4 percent of men. Gender-specific HIV prevention methods are needed but will be challenging.

HIV/AIDS-RELATED KNOWLEDGE, ATTITUDES, BELIEFS, AND BEHAVIORS

HIV Transmission

Survey research has documented that, contrary to popular belief, Mexican migrant laborers have considerable knowledge about the major modes of HIV transmission (e.g., blood, unprotected sex) (Organista et al., 1996; Organista et al., 1997a). However, they simultaneously hold many misconceptions about contracting HIV from casual modes such as mosquito bites, public bathrooms, kissing on the mouth, being coughed on, giving blood, etc. For example, a full 50 percent of the 501 migrant laborers surveyed by Organista et al. (1997a) believed that they could contract HIV from the HIV test.

Condom Knowledge and Use

The safer sex strategy of carrying and using condoms is particularly relevant to migrant laborers given their mobility and frequent geographical isolation. Unfortunately, research reveals poor condom knowledge and inconsistent use. For example, Organista et al. (1997b) found that between half and two-thirds of their sample answered either incorrectly or "don't know" to questions such as "Is Vaseline a good lubricant for condoms?" or "Should you unroll a condom before putting on penis?" When condoms are used by Mexican migrants, they are used far more often with secondary or occasional sex partners as compared to primary sex partners.

In presurvey focus groups, the following reasons were given for not using condoms with intimate, regular sex partners: It would suggest infidelity, female partner already using (nonbarrier) birth control, couple's desire to have children, etc. Consequently, only 21 percent of sexually active migrants reported "always" using condoms with regular sex partners, during the past year, as compared to 71 percent with secondary sex partners (Organista et al., 1997b). Condom promotion strategies need to consider condom use with different types of sex partners.

> I took the AIDS test because I used a woman two years ago that was a heroin addict and I started to worry about that. The problem is that, well you know, one is a man and well your needs, right? Then the opportunity presents itself for ten dollars. And at times one doesn't use any protection. I was very drunk when I used this woman.

Predictors of Condom Use

Because condom use is low and inconsistent in Mexican migrant laborers, it is important to study correlates or predictors of condom use when it does occur. Analyses of data from the previously mentioned pilot survey of eighty-seven Mexican migrant laborers revealed that condom use with both occasional and regular sex partners, as well as carrying condoms, were all predicted by procondom social norms or the perception that friends carry and use condoms (Organista et al., 1997b). Pilot study findings also showed that condom use was predicted by perceived susceptibility to contracting HIV/AIDS.

Predictors of condom use were also analyzed in the larger follow-up survey of 501 Mexican migrant laborers (Organista et al., 2000). In addition to replicating the pilot predictor study, this larger sample allowed exploration of a wide variety of sociopsychological variables while controlling for demographic and lifestyle variables well-known in the AIDS literature for their influence on condom use (e.g., age, gender, education, marital status, number of sex partners, etc.). For example, we examined "condom efficacy" which refers to how confident respondents feel about negotiating condom use with sex partners in a variety of challenging situations (e.g., subjects were asked how capable they would be of insisting on condom use if a prospective sex partner were to: get angry, not want to use a condom, threaten to leave, etc.). This variable was studied because previous research on U.S. Latinos showed that it predicts condom use with occasional sex partners (Marin, Gomez, and Tschann, 1993). Results revealed interesting patterns of predictors for the three types of condom use assessed.

Condom Use with Occasional Sex Partners

As can be seen in Table 5.1, condom use with occasional sex partners was predicted by condom efficacy and carrying condoms. All other predictors examined were nonsignificant including procondom social norms. Thus, efficacy to use condoms and keeping them handy may be central factors in condom use with occasional sex partners in Mexican migrants whose work-related lifestyles accentuate this primary HIV exposure category. For example, 82 percent of single men and 27 percent of married men in the survey reported multiple sex partners during the past year (Organista et al., 1997a).

Condom Use with Regular Sex Partners

Condom use with regular sex partners was also predicted by condom efficacy and carrying condoms in addition to positive attitudes

TABLE 5.1. Predictors of Three Types of Condom Use in Mexican Migrant Laborers (N = 501)

Condom Use with Occasional Sex Partners	Condom Use with Regular Sex Partners	Carrying Condoms
Condom efficacy	Condom efficacy	Condom efficacy
Carrying condoms	Carrying condoms	Positive condom attitudes
	Positive condoms attitudes	Procondom social norms
		Perceived susceptibility

Note: Predictors tested were: condom efficacy, procondom social norms, frequency of carrying condoms, HIV/AIDS knowledge, positive attitudes about condoms, perceived susceptibility to contracting HIV/AIDS (worry about contracting HIV/AIDS, personally know person with HIV/AIDS); and the following demographic and lifestyle control variables: number of sex partners (past year), level of acculturation, years living/working in the United States, age, gender, marital status, and education.

Source: Organista et al. (2000).

toward condoms (i.e., low belief in the following: condoms decrease sexual pleasure, interfere with sex, cause the man to lose erection, etc.). Thus, for migrants to increase their condom use in presumably intimate, ongoing sexual relationships, it appears that they must feel both efficacious and positive regarding condoms and must also keep them readily available.

Carrying Condoms

Interestingly, the seemingly simple act of carrying condoms was the most multidetermined condom-related behavior assessed, suggesting that promoting this complex behavior may be a crucial first step requiring attention to many different factors. That is, carrying condoms was predicted by condom efficacy, positive condom attitudes, procondom social norms, and perceived susceptibility to contracting HIV/AIDS. Thus, promoting carrying condoms may need to address all four of these influential predictor factors. For example, perceived susceptibility can be increased by informing Mexican migrants of their status as a new high-risk group. All three of the other predictors could be addressed by involving Mexican migrants in condom promotion efforts (e.g., communicating positive attitudes toward condoms, normalizing and endorsing condom use, and role-playing how to insist on condom use in challenging sexual situations).

CONTEXTUALIZING HIV RISK

The previously mentioned qualitative interviews began with broad questions about the life of a farmworker, how such work affects family and personal relationships, love life, and then progressed to more specific questions about risk factors.

The Experience of Migratory Labor

Farmworkers describe migratory labor as both extremely difficult and as an opportunity to work and advance beyond opportunity structures in Mexico. There is also a sense of uncertainty and apprehension with regard to the possibility of losing one's self in the United States and succumbing to *vicios* (vices) such as alcohol and drugs:

> Yes I miss my family but at the same time that I'm sacrificing, they are also sacrificing because from here I am sending [money]. I thank God and the United States that I have been sending them [money] continuously. Right now I have two girls here, one in Chicago and the other in Los Angeles. Yes, they are now citizens, so thanks to all of this, they were able to come here. They married men here, thanks to all of that.

> One can become ruined [in the United States]. One can become ruined because well the vice, the vice, the vice is very bad, whatever vice one has is bad.

Disrupted Family and Social Life

Migratory labor is described as involving the "sacrifice" of normal family relationships and friendships, resulting in frequent loneliness and susceptibility to risky behaviors:

> Sometimes I feel sad and lonely and sometimes I sit by the side of the road out there and I buy some quarts of beer and there I

am, just thinking about how they [family] are doing over there [in Mexico].

The loneliness and worry depicted in this quote reflect a susceptibility in migrant men to depression and anxiety disorders, in addition to the aforementioned alcohol and substance use disorders. For example, Alderete et al. (2000) found that male and female farmworkers had similarly high lifetime prevalence rates of mood disorders (7.2 percent and 6.7 percent, respectively) and anxiety disorders (15.1 percent and 12.9 percent, respectively) in their psychiatric prevalence study. This gender pattern contradicts general population studies that consistently show greater mood and anxiety disorders in women rather than men.

Disrupted Love and Sex Life

Although a minority of male farmworkers bring their wives and children to work in the United States, most spend months and even years away from relations in Mexico. These men are deprived of normal intimate relationships, including sex. Single as well as married men respond in a number of ways to their intimacy and sexual deprivation, such as courting available female farmworkers, whom they describe as *limpia* or "clean" with respect to STDs and HIV.

> She's a farmworker too from over there [Mexico]. We still date and we get along well. When we feel like making love, and if I have some pennies, we'll go to a hotel or even in the fields but out there where no one can see us. We get along well and that's what I do because I never got another women like those who walk the streets.

CONCEPTUAL MODEL OF RISK

Based on this research, a conceptual model of HIV risk in Mexican migrant laborers is presented here to help guide prevention and treatment strategies that are responsive to the social and cultural ecology of this complex problem area. The predominant ecological-systems perspective in social work is helpful in attempting to visualize the context of a problem and in mapping out relevant problem levels and interacting human systems. As can be seen in Figure 5.1, HIV risk in Mexican migrant laborers is first framed within the overlapping macro-level contexts of farmwork in the United States and Mexican culture. Salient dimensions of these two large contexts, pertinent to HIV risk, are then listed. For example, farmwork is characterized by mostly negative descriptors related to compromised health and well-being (e.g., hazardous, disruptive to social life, poverty, lacking in protective health policies, etc.).

Mexican culture is characterized by a mix of traditional values, norms, and role prescriptions that interact with working and living in the United States in ways related to risk. For example, Mexican constructions of sexuality that do not label a heterosexual man as homosexual, even though he may occasionally have sex with other men, need to be understood when fashioning prevention messages for different subgroups of farmworkers (Carrier, 1995). The central value of familism is another dimension of Mexican culture that needs to be studied in relation to HIV risk. For example, unaccompanied men from Mexico frequently rely on existing migration networks to relocate with relatives or other workers from the same Mexican village. Such supportive kinship networks probably reduce risk and could be incorporated into risk-reduction strategies.

Increasing numbers of indigenous farmworkers come from Mexican states such as Oaxaca, Chiapas, and Guerrero. Such individuals frequently speak more Indian dialects than Spanish and will need to be involved in reducing HIV.

Within the overlapping macro-level contexts of HIV risk are interacting micro- and meso-level factors divided into three domains: (1) farmworker subgroups (e.g., groupings by age, gender, sexual orientation, migration stream networks, etc.); (2) HIV risk behaviors (e.g., unprotected sex with prostitutes or between men or with a high-risk partner, alcohol and substance use, etc.); and (3) situational factors (e.g., drinking/drug use alone or with friends, interactions with prostitutes, men seeking men for sex, etc.). These three domains allow tailored interventions to the target population by focusing on different farmworker subgroups by risk behavior by situation interactions. For example, an intervention focusing on adult male migrants by unprotected sex with prostitutes by alcohol/drug use in bars is highly warranted in view of the literature reviewed. Another focus

OVERLAPPING MACRO-LEVEL CONTEXTS

MIGRANT LABOR IN UNITED STATES

Opportunity to progress

Difficult work
— labor intensive
— hazardous
— exploitative

Lack of legal protection
— health and safety standards
— employee benefits

Poverty inducing
— low-paying work
— inconsistent work
— substandard housing

Disrupts social life
— marital/family/friends
— loneliness

Changes love and sex life
— intimacy deprivation
— sexual deprivation
— more sexual freedom

Barriers to services
— scarce
— culturally unresponsive
— ineligibility

Increases vulnerability to risk

MEXICAN CULTURE

Spanish language

Familism

Traditional gender roles
— machismo
— marianismo

Constructions of (homo)sexuality

Personalism

Sexual silence and conservatism

Catholicism

INTERACTING MICRO- AND MESO-LEVEL FACTORS

Subgroups of Migrant Laborers	Situational Factors	Risk Behaviors
Farmworkers — seasonal — permanent	*Drinking/drug use* — alone — with co-workers	*Unprotected sex* — with prostitutes — between men — with high-risk partner
Urban-based — service sector — day laborers	*Interacting with prostitutes* — on the street — at bars (straight, gay, transgender) — at work site	*Alcohol and substance use*
Adult men	*Men seeking men for sex* — casual/romantic — sex for money/drugs — between same/different sexual orientations	*Needle sharing* — illicit drugs — therapeutic injections
Adult women		
Adolescents		
Men who have sex with men (MSM) — gay — straight — etc.		
IDU		

FIGURE 5.1. Conceptual Model of HIV Risk in Mexican Migrant Laborers

could be on the interaction between gay-identified farmworkers by unprotected sex with co-workers.

IMPLICATIONS FOR HIV PREVENTION AND TREATMENT SERVICES: STATE OF THE ART AND BEYOND

Problematic State of the Art

HIV Prevention

Currently, a loose network of public and private, government and nonprofit, health and social service programs provide minimal HIV prevention and even less AIDS treatment services to Mexican migrant laborers in the United States. As either part of larger agencies or separate entities, such programs typically deliver HIV/AIDS services within a broader array of health and social services. Highly dedicated frontline staff reach amazing numbers of people, despite meager agency resources, usually through an outreach model in which trusted bilingual and bicultural service providers (many from migrant labor backgrounds themselves) reach migrants where they live and work.

Prevention services typically consist of basic "HIV 101" education, condom distribution, and information about available related services. For example, in a review of 181 California agencies providing HIV/AIDS services to Latino communities, Castañeda and Collins (1997) report the following rates and types of most common services: 93 percent HIV/AIDS education, 52 percent counseling/ therapy to HIV-positive clients, 49 percent HIV testing, and 49 percent support groups for HIV-positive clients.

These HIV/AIDS services are explicitly and implicitly based upon the health beliefs model (HBM) which posits that risk reduction is a function of: (1) belief that a disease is serious; (2) perception of self as susceptible to the disease; and (3) belief that taking action to decrease susceptibility will be helpful (Rosenstock, Strecher, and Becker, 1988). Unfortunately, applications of the HBM to HIV prevention have produced mixed results across different (nonmigrant) groups and risk factors (for brief review see McBride et al., 1999). In fact, agency staff are usually aware that HIV/AIDS education misses the multi-determined complexity of risk behaviors and that we must develop, implement, and evaluate approaches that conceptualize HIV risk in ways responsive to the work and culture-related realities of Mexican migrant laborers.

General Recommendations for Improving HIV/AIDS Services

A few general and gender-specific recommendations are in order before discussing more innovative approaches to HIV prevention with Mexican migrant laborers (Balls Organista and Organista, 1997). Because there are virtually no studies in the literature of AIDS treatment programs for farmworkers, the main emphasis should be on HIV prevention. Discussion of programs should include attention to theory and values, implementation, criticisms, and review of effectiveness where possible.

Basic HIV/AIDS information must be communicated to Mexican farmworkers in Spanish (e.g., 81 percent of our large survey sample spoke only or mostly Spanish), and written literature must be geared to the appropriate reading level (average years of education equals four to seven in survey sample). HIV prevention outreach must be done where migrants live and work (e.g., labor camps), and the delivery of intervention messages should probably be done separately for men and women given the sexual conservativism of traditional Mexican people (de la Vega, 1990). As mentioned earlier, indigenous Mexican migrants will need to be increasingly involved in HIV prevention efforts with similar groups of workers.

Migrant Men

Condom promotion efforts with male Mexican farmworkers must include basic instructions on proper condom use including "hands-on" practice with phallic replicas. Men should be urged to carry or keep condoms handy in the spirit of being *hombres preparados* (prepared men), a term that carries the connotation of being learned in addition to prepared. HIV transmission with different types of sex partners should be discussed. For example, the common practice of using prostitutes while in the United States, including the occasional practice of the *hermanos de leche* ritual, should be addressed in detail. Can men still be *hermanos de leche* if condoms are used? Isn't it important for *hermanos verdaderos* (real brothers) to protect one another? What might be some less risky forms of male bonding?

The topic of sex between men (and specifically unprotected anal sex) must not be restricted to "homosexual" men but should acknowledge the occasional participation of heterosexual or bisexual men and the need to protect their female partners by using condoms with occasional male sex partners. In a study of 190 Mexican immigrants, Mikawa et al. (1992) found that using condoms to "protect the woman" predicted condom use as opposed to using condoms to protect one's own health. This finding appears to reflect the value of machismo in the positive sense of protecting the well-being of women.

Because of the apparent central role of condom efficacy in predicting condom use with secondary sex partners, sufficient discussion and role-playing should be used to practice insistence on condom use in challenging sexual situations frequently encountered by Mexican male migrants (e.g., encountering prostitutes in bars while drinking with encouraging co-workers on payday).

Female Partners of Male Migrants

Female migrants in our surveys were extremely low in acculturation and thus presumably high in traditional Mexican culture and adherence to conservative gender roles (Balls Organista, Organista, and Soloff, 1999; Organista et al., 1997a). Working within traditional gender roles could involve urging Mexican women to protect themselves in order to prevent the congenital transmission of HIV to children. Similarly, because Mexican women are central to their family's health and well-being, they could be reminded to protect their own health for the sake of their family. However, working outside of traditional Mexican culture is also needed and may not be as difficult as often presumed given the changing nature of gender roles, especially in migrant and immigrant women. Amaro (1988) has advocated the use of focus groups with Latinas in which discussions would focus on their beliefs about realistic and effective prevention strategies.

Innovative Approaches to HIV Prevention

Empowering Health Circles

Magaña et al. (1992) have advocated the use of *circulos de salud* (health circles) for HIV prevention with Latinos based on the empowering and progressive work of Brazilian educator Paulo Freire. Theoretically, Freire maintained that oppressed groups can only truly improve their lives by generating their own definitions and solutions to problems that affect them. Furthermore, problem definitions and solutions generated by professionals or agents of the establishment will inevitably perpetuate the status quo for oppressed groups, even if well-intentioned.

With regard to HIV prevention, Magaña et al. (1992) advocate health circles that begin by providing participants with basic information about HIV transmission and prevention, but then involve the participants in an active problem-solving discussion after posing relevant risky situations. No evaluation or feasibility analysis has been applied to this model but it is consistent with the recommendations of service providers and researchers to actively involve farmworkers in all stages of HIV/AIDS program development and implementation (Connor, Mishra, and Magaña, 1996).

Chicano Theater

The *Teatro Campesino* (Farmworker Theater) is a Chicano theater company that is occasionally active in the area of HIV prevention by writing and delivering *actos* (brief plays) to campesinos dealing with HIV/AIDS. The Teatro Campesino is a distinctly politicized and entertaining Chicano art medium with street theater roots in 1960s when it was created to educate and activate farmworker involvement in labor issues (e.g., Cesar Chavez' United Farmworker Union). In addition to delivering humorous and dramatic plays to where farmworkers live and work, members of the farmworker audience have been frequently invited into the actos to act out their lived experiences. The idea of using this conceptual model, as well as relevant research, to inform workers about HIV prevention, complete with an evaluation piece, is an intriguing one that researchers in California should pursue.

Condom Promotion with Prostitutes

In a rare empirical study, Mishra and Conner (1996) evaluated the effectiveness of an intervention designed to increase condom use with prostitutes, as well as to improve HIV/AIDS-related knowledge and attitudes, among 193 Mexican male farmworkers in Southern California. Participants were provided with HIV prevention information in the culture-based form of Mexican style *fotonovelas* (photo novellas). *Radionovelas* (radio novellas) were also broadcasted daily on a local Spanish language station and participants were given radios, program times, and encouraged to tune in. The *novelas* depicted three scenarios in which a male farmworker respectively: (1) uses a condom with a prostitute; (2) abstains from sex with the prostitute; (3) infects wife and child with HIV as a result of unprotected sex with the prostitute.

All participants were pre- and posttested and results showed significant gains in HIV/AIDS knowledge and related attitudes, and in reported condom use with prostitutes. Of those men who used prostitutes during the course of the study, twenty of thirty-seven reported condom use after participation in the study versus one of thirty-two prior to participation. This study demonstrates the promise of using culture and farmwork-sensitive methods to target a particular farmworker subgroup (adult men) by risk factor (unprotected sex) by situation (sex with prostitute) interaction. With regard to theoretical underpinnings, this program appeared to tap at least two areas in a culturally sensitive manner: increasing perceived susceptibility (to self and family); and promoting procondom social norms among male farmworkers via role modeling of similar others in the novelas.

Peer Education to Men Who Have Sex with Men (MSM)

In San Jose, California, the Health Education and Training Center (HETC), Inc., and the Mexican American Community Services Agency (MACSA) have been collaborating on an extraordinary peer education program. Latino male-to-female transvestite and transgendered peers are trained to deliver HIV prevention messages to migrant men who have sex with men, and in gay Latino bars where these peers perform nighttime entertainment shows (i.e., dancing, singing, impersonations).

Many weeks were invested in gaining access to the bars and earning the trust of the *las muchachas* (the girls), as the peers refer to themselves. Afterward, the girls received training and developed ways of integrating HIV prevention information into their bar shows. This Spanish language, indigenous, and subculture-based style of program delivery is both humorous and entertaining (e.g., impersonations of well-known actresses from Spanish language television *novelas,* etc.). In one recent skit, a Monica Lewinsky impersonator, complete with blue stained dress, is scorned for not having used a condom on President Clinton as a way of avoiding the stain and subsequent *locura* (craziness).

The peers were motivated to participate by the dual desire to help the Latino community and to meet as a support group convened by HETC staff. Transvestite and transgendered Latinos are even more marginalized than gay and lesbian Latinos within the Latino community and as a result have their own unique set of risk factors and pressing needs.

With regard to theory, the peer education program claims to follow the stages of change theory (Prochaska, DiClemente, and Norcross, 1992) which posits that individuals move through a series of stages of readiness in the adoption of health-promoting behaviors and cessation of risk behaviors:

1. *pre-contemplation* refers to not considering behavior change in near future (i.e., during the next six months);
2. *contemplation* refers to awareness of personal risk and intention to change in near future;
3. *preparation* refers to intention to take action within the immediate future (e.g., one month);
4. *action* stage refers to when an individual has made lifestyle changes during the past six months; and
5. *maintenance* refers to successful lifestyle changes during the past six months and the need to focus on relapse prevention.

The staff at HETC claim to continually assess what stage their target group is at by conducting periodic interviews and focus groups with key informants (e.g., participants, service providers, gatekeepers, etc.). Strategies to move groups from precontemplation to contemplation include heightening awareness of risk and prochange values.

The action stage is prompted through persuasion, motivation, and problem solving around obstacles to change.

Although attention to theory is to be applauded in the peer education program, there is most likely significant individual variation within the target group, with respect to stages of change, that may not be best addressed by the group-level assessment and intervention methods described. With regard to program evaluation, the peer education program is not unusual in its lack of resources and personnel to empirically assess changes in risk behaviors.

Top-Down Government-Sponsored Prevention Programs

Recent work by Haour-Knipe, Fleury, and Dubois-Arber (1999) has documented an impressive government-sponsored HIV/AIDS prevention program for migrant laborers in Switzerland. The Swiss Migrant Project is part of the country's National AIDS Plan and is designed to target urban-based Turkish, Portugese, and Spanish migrants that work in the hotel and construction industries nine out of twelve months during the year.

Through a comprehensive, top-down collaboration between public health officials and nongovernment organizations, project structure and staffing were developed at the migrant community level by involving program coordinators and peer educators charged with designing culturally specific HIV/AIDS prevention strategies. In terms of planning, the first phase of the program consisted of exploratory studies to gauge the needs of migrant communities as well as recruitment of program staff. The second phase involved the establishment of various flexible community-level programs complete with process evaluation. The final phase involved the formal implementation of refined programs complete with program evaluation. Results showed successful utilization of local community programs by migrants as well as HIV/AIDS-related knowledge, attitudes, and risk behaviors comparable to the general Swiss public.

Although HIV risk assessment was slim in the Swiss Migrant Project (e.g., condom use with a casual sex partner), it does demonstrate the feasibility, need, and promise of placing migrant HIV prevention within a national HIV prevention plan. Acceptance of government involvement was won by involving members of the migrant community in local program development and delivery aimed at hard-to-reach and hidden high-risk groups, sometimes outside of official government jurisdiction (e.g., undocumented workers).

With regard to HIV/AIDS treatment, Haour-Knipe, Fleury, and Dubois-Arber (1999) noted the frustration of community workers that occasionally encountered migrants with HIV/AIDS. There were simply no official ways of helping given the program's prevention mission and design. Certainly, services to HIV/AIDS-affected migrants is a logical next step.

LONG-TERM RECOMMENDATIONS: EXPANDING RESOURCES, INFRASTRUCTURE, AND LABOR REFORM

According to Harthorn (1998), farmworker interventions that change microscopic effects of the global economy, agricultural business, and policies may be of limited value. This assertion highlights the importance of contextualizing farmworker problems within their multiple human systems and ecological levels. The HIV prevention programs reviewed and recommended generally involved micro- and meso-level interventions, at the community level, which are responsive to Mexican culture and the experience of migratory labor. Certainly, greater attention to macro-level social and political forces is needed to influence policy.

Building Upon Community-Based Services

In Castañeda and Collins' (1997) survey of 181 California agencies that provide HIV/AIDS prevention services to Latinos, they generally found that community-based organizations (CBOs) were more effective than federal and state agencies because of their greater number of bilingual staff, volunteers, and culturally sensitive approaches to service delivery. Although the Latino-focused agencies in the study were fewer and smaller than non-Latino-focused agencies, they had more bilingual/bicultural staff, less staff turnover, made greater use of Spanish media, and provided more one-on-one HIV/AIDS services. However, it was also found that non-Latino-focused agencies provided more services to farmworkers because there were no Latino-focused agencies in rural, small-town communities.

Findings from this study indicate the need to extend and build upon the existing network of community and migrant health centers including community-based, Latino-focused agencies providing HIV/ AIDS services. Such a direction needs to involve expanding the network of centers, increasing and consolidating multiple social and health services within these centers, increasing collaborations between CBOs and researchers to develop and evaluate local programs, and continuing to advocate for equal protection of farmworkers under the law.

Expanding the Network of Community and Migrant Health Centers

According to Blumenthal, Lukomnik, and Hawkins (1993), there are about 580 federally funded and 500 nonfederally funded community and migrant health centers that serve predominantly poor, ethnic-minority, and underserved clientele. Those who use these services show better health than nonusers at about one-third the cost per patient as compared to the national average. In fact, Blumenthal, Lukomnik, and Hawkins (1993) note that only one-third of 1 percent of federal health expenditures go to these centers. The majority of clients at these centers are among the nation's uninsured (estimated at between 31 and 37 million) and/or reside in rural and urban settings extremely short of health care professionals (estimated at about 34 million). The number of these centers should be tripled nationally (i.e., to about 3,000) in order to meet the basic health needs of these groups at a cost of only about 1 percent of federal health expenditures.

Consolidation and Coordination of Services

Napolitano and Goldberg (1998) advocate the coordination and integration of a broad array of employment, social, legal, and medical services for farmworkers. Such a system would also need to include the creation of a centralized database of farmworker medical records and the consolidation of services at accessible sites. At the national level, Martin and Martin (1994) advocate the creation of an interagency council to coordinate the "big four" federal assistant programs for migrant farmworkers: Migrant Health, Migrant Education, Migrant Head Start, and job training. They note that for a three-year period, beginning in 1984, Migrant Health and Migrant Education were authorized to coordinate their services to better meet the overlapping health and educational needs of migrant farmworker children and families. Martin and Martin (1994) also advocate long-term improvements in immigration and labor laws in the direction of reforming agricultural labor conditions and decreasing competition for farmwork through stricter reinforcement of immigration laws (e.g., reducing number of undocumented in order to promote a more politically powerful workforce).

Collaborative Research

The literature includes more suggestions on how researchers and CBO staff can codevelop, implement, and evaluate HIV prevention programs aimed at hard-to-reach and hidden high-risk groups. For example, Schensul (1999) recommends the following guidelines:

1. building trust via multiple site visits and securing needed funds to support research;
2. beginning with modest studies that help to better understand the target populations, and which assess the feasibility of pilot intervention programs (large efficacy studies can follow depending on success);
3. continuously and flexibly negotiate everyone's role in the research project with attention to differences and overlap in the team's research and direct service needs.

Without a research arm, we cannot expect CBOs to pursue empirical program evaluation, and without start-up monies, we cannot expect to engage CBOs in collaboration.

The Need to Amend Federal Laws That Are Hazardous to Farmworker Health

Farm and nonfarm labor parity under the law, and equal protection of farmworker health, safety, and economic well-being, will require major amendments to federal and state laws and policies. Simply put, if farmworkers are essential to the multibillion-dollar agricultural sector of the U.S. economy, then they deserve the same labor rights and protection as American workers. There is no ethical justification in exploiting farmworkers' labor and placing their health at far greater risk than their American counterparts, simply because they are predominantly poor, Mexican noncitizens, and frequently undocumented. Inclusion of farmworkers in federal laws such as the 1935 National Labor Relations Act, the 1938 Fair Labor Standards Act, and the 1970 Occupational Safety and Health Act would improve farmworkers' wages, employee benefits, and health- and safety-related working conditions. According to Sakala (1987), work-related deaths, injuries, disabilities, and related illnesses need to be treated as part of the cost of production, just as they are elsewhere in American labor, and paid for by some combination of employer and federal government funding. Only then will significant improvements in farmworkers' health, including decreased risk for HIV/AIDS, be realized.

REFERENCES

Alderete, E., Vega, W. A., Kolody, B., and Aguilar-Gaxiola, S. (2000). Lifetime prevalence of risk factors for psychiatric disorders among Mexican migrant farmworkers in California. *American Journal of Public Health, 90*(4), 608-614.

Amaro, H. (1988). Considerations for prevention of HIV infection among Hispanic women. *Psychology of Women Quarterly, 12,* 429-443.

Balls Organista, P. and Organista, K. C. (1997). Culture and gender sensitive AIDS prevention with Mexican migrant laborers: A primer for counselors. *Journal of Multicultural Counseling and Development, 25,* 121-129.

Balls Organista, P., Organista, K. C., and Soloff, P. R. (1998). Exploring AIDS-related knowledge, attitudes, and behaviors of female Mexican migrant workers. *Health and Social Work, 23*(2), 81-160.

Blackmore, C. A., Limpakarnjanarat, K., Rigau-Perez, J. G., Albritton, W. L., and Greenwood, J. R. (1985). An outbreak of chancroid in Orange County, California: Descriptive epidemiology and disease-control measures. *Journal of Infectious Diseases, 151*(5), 840-844.

Blumenthal, D. S., Lukomnik, J. E., and Hawkins, D. R. Jr. (1993). A proposal to provide care to the uninsured through a network of community health centers. *Journal of Health Care for the Poor and Underserved, 4*(3), 273-279.

Bronfman, M. and Minello, N. (1992). *Habitos sexuales de los migrantes temporales Mexicanos a los Estados Unidos de America, practicas de riesgo para la infección por VIH* [Sexual habits of seasonal Mexican migrants to the United States of America, risk practices for HIV infection]. Mexico, DF: El Colegio de Mexico.

Carrier, J. (1995). *De los otros [of the others]: Intimacy and homosexuality among Mexican men.* New York: Columbia University Press.

Carrier, J. M. and Magaña, J. R. (1991). Use of ethnosexual data on men of Mexican origin for HIV/AIDS prevention programs. *The Journal of Sex Research, 28,* 189-202.

Castañeda, D. and Collins, B. E. (1997). Structure and activities of agencies providing HIV and AIDS education and prevention to Latino/a communities. *AIDS Education and Prevention, 9*(6), 533-550.

Centers for Disease Control (1988). HIV seroprevalence in migrant and seasonal farmworkers—North Carolina, 1987. *Morbidity and Mortality Weekly Report, 37*(34), 517-519.

Connor, R. F., Mishra, S. I., and Magaña, R. (1996). HIV prevention policies and programs: Perspectives from researchers, migrant workers, and policymakers. In S. I. Mishra, R. F. Connor, and J. R. Magaña (Eds.), *AIDS crossing borders: The spread of HIV among migrant laborers* (pp.185-214). Boulder, CO: Westview Press.

de la Vega, E. (1990). Considerations for reaching the Latino population with sexuality and HIV/AIDS information and education. *Siecus Report, 18*(3), 1-8.

Decosas, J., Kane F., Anarfi, J. K., Sodii, K. D. R., and Wagner, H. U. (1995). Migration and AIDS. *Lancet, 346,* 826-828.

Department of Labor (1990). *An atlas of state profiles which estimate number of migrant and seasonal farmworkers and members of their families.* Washington, DC: Office of Migrant Health.

Haour-Knipe, M., Fleury, F., and Dubois-Arber, F. (1999). HIV/AIDS prevention for migrants and ethnic minorities: Three phase evaluation. *Social Science and Medicine, 49,* 1357-1372.

Harthorn, B. H. (1998). California farmworkers: Dilemmas in developing interventions for health and medical care concerns. *Human Organization, 57*(3), 369-378.

Hulewicz, J. M. (1994). AIDS knows no borders. *World AIDS, 35,* 6-10.

Inciardi, J. A., Surratt, H. L., Colon, H. M., Chitwood, D. D., and Rivers, J. E. (1999). Drug use and HIV risk among migrant workers on the Delmarva Peninsula. *Substance Use and Misuse, 34*(4 and 5), 653-666.

Jochelson, K., Mothibeli, M., and Leger, J. (1994). Human immunodeficiency virus and migrant labor in south Africa. In N. Krieger and M. Glenn (Eds.), *AIDS: Politics of survival* (pp. 141-160). Amityville, NY: Baywood Publishing Company.

Lafferty, J. (1991). Self-injection and needle sharing among migrant farmworkers. *American Journal of Public Health, 81,* 221.

López, R. and Ruiz, J. D. (1995). Seroprevalence of human immunodeficiency virus type I and syphilis and assessment of risk behaviors among migrant and seasonal farmworkers in Northern California. Manuscript prepared for Office of AIDS, California Department of Health Services.

Magaña, J. R. (1991). Sex, drugs and HIV: An ethnographic approach. *Social Science and Medicine, 33,* 5-9.

Magaña, J. R., Ferreira-Pinto, J. B., Blair, M., and Mata, A. Jr. (1992). Una pedagogia de concientizacion para la prevencion del VIH/SIDA. [A pedagogy of conscientization for the prevention of HIV/AIDS]. *Revista Latino Americana De Psicologia* [Latin American Journal of Psychology], *24*(1-2), 97-108.

Marin, B. V., Gomez, C., and Tschann, J. M. (1993). Condom use among Hispanic men with multiple female partners: A nine-state study. *Public Health Reports, 25,* 742-750.

Martin, P. L. and Martin, D. A. (1994). *The endless quest: Helping America's farmworkers.* Boulder, CO: Westview Press.

McBride, D. C., Weatherby, N. L., Inciardi, J. A., and Gillespite, S. A. (1999). AIDS susceptibility in a migrant population: Perception and behavior. *Substance Use and Misuse, 34*(4 and 5), 633-652.

McVea, K. L. S. P. (1997). Lay injection practices among migrant farmworkers in the age of AIDS: Evolution of biomedical folk practices. *Social Science and Medicine, 45*(1), 91-98.

Mikawa, J. K., Morones, P. A., Gomez, A., Case, H. L., Olsen, D., and Gonzales-Huss, M. J. (1992). Cultural practices of Hispanics: Implications for the prevention of AIDS. *Hispanic Journal of the Behavioral Sciences, 14*(4), 421-433.

Mines, R., Gabbard, S., and Steirman, A. (1997). *A profile of U.S. farmworkers: Demographics, household composition, income and use of services.* Washington, DC: Office of Program Economics, Office of the Assistant Secretary for Policy, U.S. Department of Labor; Research Report No. 6, prepared for the Commission on Immigration Reform.

Mines, R., Mullenax, N., and Saca, L. (2001). *The binational farmworker health survey: An in-depth study of agricultral worker health in Mexico and the United States.* Davis, CA: California Institute for Rural Studies.

Mishra, S. I. and Conner, R. F. (1996). Evaluation of an HIV prevention program among Latino farmworkers. In S. I. Mishra, R. F. Connor, and J. R. Magaña (Eds.), *AIDS crossing borders: The spread of HIV among migrant Latinos* (pp. 157-181). Boulder, CO: Westview Press.

Moses, M. (1993). Farmworkers and pesticides. In R. D. Bullard (Ed.), *Confronting environmental racism: Voices from the grassroots* (pp. 161–178). Boston: South End Press.

Napolitano, M. and Goldberg, B. W. (1998). Migrant health. In S. Loue (Ed.), *Handbook of immigrant health* (pp. 261-276). New York: Plenum Press.

National Advisory Council on Migrant Health (1995). *Losing ground: The condition of farmworkers in America.* Bethesda, MD: Department of Health and Human Services/Health Resources and Services Administration, Bureau of Primary Health Care, Migrant Health Branch.

Organista, K. C. and Balls Organista, P. (1997). Migrant laborers and AIDS in the United States: A review of the literature. *AIDS Education and Prevention, 9,* 83-93.

Organista, K. C., Balls Organista, P., Bola, J., Garcia de Alba, G. J. E., and Castillo Moran, M. A. (2000). Predictors of condom use in Mexican migrant laborers. *American Journal of Community Psychology, 28*(2), 245-265.

Organista, K. C., Balls Organista, P., Garcia de Alba, G. J. E., and Castillo Moran, M. A. (1997b). Psychosocial predictors of condom use in Mexican migrant laborers. *Interamerican Journal of Psychology, 31*(1), 77-90.

Organista, K. C., Balls Organista, P., Garcia de Alba, G. J. E., Castillo Moran, M. A., and Carrillo, H. (1996). AIDS and condom-related knowledge, beliefs, and behaviors in Mexican migrant laborers. *Hispanic Journal of Behavioral Sciences, 18,* 392-406.

Organista, K. C., Balls Organista, P., Garcia de Alba, G. J. E., Castillo Moran, M. A., and Ureta Carrillo, L. E. (1997a). Survey of condom-related beliefs, behaviors, and perceived social norms in Mexican migrant laborers. *Journal of Community Health, 22*(3), 185-198.

Prochaska, J. O., DiClemente, C. C., and Norcross, J. C. (1992). In search of how people change: Applications to addictive behaviors. *American Psychologist, 47*(9), 1102-1114.

Rosenstock, I. M., Strecher, V., and Becker, M. H. (1988). Social learning theory and the health belief model. *Health Education Quarterly, 15,* 175-183.

Rust, G. S. (1990). Health status of migrants farmworkers: A literature review and commentary. *American Journal of Public Health, 80*(10), 1213-1217.

Sakala, C. (1987). Migrant and seasonal farmworkers in the United States: A review of health hazards, status, and policy. *International Migration Review, 21*(3), 659-687.

Schenker, M. B. (1996). Preventive medicine and health promotion are overdue in the agricultural work place. *Journal of Public Health Policy, 17*(3), 275-303.

Schensul, J. J. (1999). Organizing community research partnerships in the struggle against AIDS. *Health Education and Behavior, 26*(2), 266-283.

Schoonover Smith, L. (1988). Ethnic differences in knowledge of sexually transmitted diseases in North American black and Mexican-American farmworkers. *Research in Nursing and Health, 11,* 51-58.

Slesinger, D. O. (1992). Health status and needs of migrant farmworkers in the United States: A literature review. *The Journal of Rural Health, 8*(3), 227-234.

U.S. Department of Labor (1990). Findings from the National Agricultural Workers Survey (NAWS): A demographic and employment profile of perishable crop farmworkers. Washington, DC: Author.

U.S. Department of Labor (1998). Findings from the National Agricultural Workers Survey (NAWS): A demographic and employment profile of United States farmworkers. Washington, DC: Author.

Villarejo, D., Lighthall, D., Williams, D., III., Souter, A., Mines, R., Bade, B., Samuels, S., and McCurdy, S. A. (2000). *Suffering in silence: A report on the health of California's agricultural workers.* Davis, CA: California Institute for Rural Studies.

Chapter 6

A Family Intervention Model for Engaging Hidden At-Risk African Americans in HIV Prevention Programs

Larry D. Icard
Nushina Siddiqui

INTRODUCTION

Getting at-risk groups to participate in prevention programs has been a long-standing problem for HIV practitioners and researchers. Now at the end of the second decade of the HIV pandemic, health practitioners and researchers are currently faced with new challenges as they struggle to find more effective ways to involve at-risk African Americans, particularly those hidden segments of the population, in HIV prevention programs.

Twenty-three years since the discovery of HIV/AIDS, dramatic shifts have occurred among populations at high risk of infection. Cases of HIV infection in gay white men, the population most at risk during the initial years of the epidemic, have significantly declined while rates of HIV infection among African Americans have increased and continue to do so at alarming rates. Reports suggest that among African Americans, men and women with lower levels of education and income living in urban areas are most at risk (Cummings et al., 1997).

Cultural values and attitudes as well as religious beliefs become strong barriers blocking some segments of the African-American public from participating in HIV prevention programs. Of particular concern are those segments of African Americans who are likely to be stigmatized for illegal or ill-favored behaviors such as drug abuse, prostitution, and same-sex relationships. These men and women are far less likely to participate in HIV prevention programs than other segments in the African-American population. Stigmatized and marginalized African Americans are often the most elusive and hidden, and the most vulnerable to becoming infected with HIV. This chapter addresses this concern. Within this context, we discuss the merits that family-focused interventions offer health practitioners and researchers in their efforts to effectively engage hidden at-risk African Americans in HIV prevention programs.

A brief overview of the epidemiology of HIV infection among African Americans is discussed first. Against this backdrop, the definition of hidden segments within the African-American population is further articulated. The discussion then shifts to highlight the salient characteristics and common features of family-focused HIV interventions. Following an overview of family-focused interventions, the chapter discusses factors to consider for designing family-focused HIV interventions to help engage hidden segments of at-risk African Americans, specifically adult African-American men and women. The chapter concludes with a summary of the strengths, limitations, and future directions for using family-focused interventions to engage hidden segments of high-risk African Americans in HIV prevention programs.

AFRICAN AMERICANS AND HIV

Although comprising 13 percent of the U.S. population, African Americans account for nearly half of all new AIDS cases (CDC, 2001a). AIDS is the fourth leading cause of death among African Americans ages twenty-five to forty-four. African-American women comprise 64 percent of new AIDS cases among women (CDC, 2001a). Injection drug use accounts for 41 percent of all AIDS cases among African-American women since the epidemic began, and 38 percent are attributed to heterosexual contact (CDC, 2002). In addition to the direct risks of infection associated with drug injection (sharing needles), drug use is fueling the heterosexual spread of the epidemic; a large proportion of women are infected through sex with an injection drug user. In light of this fact, engaging the drug-using population and their sexual partners in prevention programs continues to be one of the priorities for HIV prevention researchers and practitioners.

Current reports show that 79 percent of people with AIDS in the United States are men; of these, 41 percent were infected through male-to-male sex. Of new cases of AIDS among men, African-American men comprise 39 percent. African-American men who have sex with men (MSM) are more likely than their white counterparts to engage in high-risk activities and to be HIV infected (Diaz, Ayala, and Bein, 1999). Social and cultural factors may limit the ability of African-American MSM to protect themselves from HIV (Stokes and Peterson, 1998). Valleroy et al. (2000), investigating the current state of the HIV epidemic among adolescent and young adult MSM, found that the prevalence of HIV is higher among blacks (14.1 percent) than Hispanics (6.9 percent) and whites (3.3 percent).

The rate of HIV infection among incarcerated African-American men is of additional concern. Nearly 10,000 confirmed AIDS cases are in federal, state, and local correctional facilities: 6,200 in state prisons, 3,100 in local jails, and 430 in federal institutions (Bureau of Justice Statistics, 1999). According to federal government reports, the proportion of male inmates with HIV (2.3 percent) is much higher than the proportion of HIV-infected males in the general population (.6 percent) (U.S. Department of Justice, 1999). Approximately 75 percent of the 2 million people in prisons and jails are Latino or African American. African Americans are almost eight times more likely to be incarcerated in local jails than whites (AIDS Action, 2001). Consequently, among the incarcerated African-American men who are released back into the general population, reports suggest that a staggering number of these men are HIV positive (Bull, 2001).

Incarcerated African-American women also comprise a population that is particularly vulnerable to HIV infection. Reports show that African-American females are eight times more likely than white women to be in prison. HIV has disproportionately impacted African-American women in recent years (CDC, 1998). To date, little is known about the etiology and epidemiology of HIV/AIDS among African-American women who have been released from incarceration. Once released, these women are likely to become hidden from conventional strategies used to engage participants in HIV prevention programs.

These observations shed light on young and adult African-American MSM, intravenous drug users, and African-American men and women released from incarceration who are at high risk of becoming infected with HIV and who are often difficult to engage in prevention programs. A closer look at some of the characteristics of these hidden populations reveals some of the concerns that family-based interventions can address to more effectively engage members of these populations in HIV prevention programs.

AFRICAN AMERICANS AS HIDDEN POPULATIONS

The term "hidden population" is commonly used to refer to populations that are elusive or difficult to access. In discussions of hidden populations, it is important to keep in mind that these populations as such are highly multifaceted, characterized by multilevel stratifications of varying levels of ostracism and degrees of marginalization. These multifarious and multileveled stratifications of groupings of hidden populations are shaped by societal norms and cultural values pertaining to the behavior in question, and the degree to which social networks of hidden populations are structured and formalized. The less coupled or formed the network, the more hidden the population. The more incongruous the behavior with the norms of general society, the more obscure and hidden the population.

Hidden populations are commonly defined by stigmatized or illegal activities such as drug use, same-sex behavior, or prostitution (Siegel et al., 1991; CDC, 1990; CDC, 1993; Metzger et al., 1993; Stewart, Zuckerman, and Inge, 1994). Notwithstanding the impact of the socially stigmatized behavior itself, factors such as cultural attitudes, religious beliefs, and poverty significantly contribute to men and women becoming hidden and unwilling to participate in HIV prevention programs. Involvement in illicit or stigmatized behavior may result in these men and women being subjected to the pressures, subjugations, and ostracizations from both the general society and the black community. For example, racism coupled with the societal prohibitions against excessive drinking and drug abuse among women can result in substance-abusing African-American women experiencing strong condemnation from the general society. These women may also experience condemnation and rejection from the black community for violating cultural gender norms (Gray and Littlefield, 2002). A number of writers have commented on the importance of racial and ethnic communities for the mental health and emotional well-being of racial or ethnic minority individuals (Gary, 1978). The potential alienation and rejection from both the black community and general society may result in some female substance abusers becoming withdrawn or furtive in their daily lives. These women are also likely to be elusive and hidden from efforts to engage them in HIV prevention programs. Developing effective ways to involve African-American men and women who are members of hidden populations is a daunting task for HIV prevention practitioners and researchers.

Among hidden populations, African-American men who are on the "down low" (DL) are particularly challenging to engage in HIV prevention efforts. African-American men on the DL are men who engage in same-sex behaviors but do not identify themselves as gay or bisexual. Poverty or harsh economic conditions may lead some African-American DL men to have sex with other men in exchange for money or other economic benefits. Cultural norms pertaining to masculinity and male behavior contribute heavily to many African-American men's decisions to wholly conceal their sexual lives. An African-American man on the DL is unlikely to go to a gay bar. His sexual encounters are often brief, with a partner he has met anonymously in a public space or possibly over the Internet. The short time that it takes him to negotiate and engage in sex leaves little time and extremely limited opportunities for health practitioners and researchers to engage him in HIV prevention programs.

Because race and sex are two of the most salient features in the construction of identity, negative attitudes toward same-sex behavior espoused by the black church can create tension between components of one's identity, thereby leaving African-American MSM who have strong identifications with church and community living what seems to be irresolvable conflicting lives. Denial may be played out through impersonal, informal sexual encounters.

Domestic abuse is another important risk criterion that warrants consideration. African-American women living in abusive relationships are another crucial at-risk hidden population. Abused women are four times more likely than nonabused women to engage in sex with a risky sexual partner (El-Bassel et al., 1999). Often, the presence of physical abuse in a relationship prevents women from asking their partners to use a condom. Abused women are also less likely to receive the social support that they require, because they must often take into consideration the threat of partner violence when making decisions about seeking social support.

Physical and sexual partner abuse and HIV infection have emerged as intersecting epidemics among inner-city African-American women. Situations in which African-American women are forced into having sex with a seropositive male partner are increasingly being reported. A couple's drug involvement also increases the risk of physical and sexual violence and concomitant sexual HIV risks (El-Bassel et al., 2000). Clearly, male dominance and control function to isolate and prevent females from accessing the support they need to cope with partner violence, thereby making them another hard-to-reach population (El-Bassel et al., 2001).

FAMILY-FOCUSED INTERVENTIONS
AND HIDDEN POPULATIONS

Many of the strategies for reaching at-risk populations are based on models developed during the early years of the HIV/AIDS epidemic. During the first decade of the HIV/AIDS epidemic, largely white gay men were affected. Because the onset of AIDS appeared on the heels of the gay rights movement, politicization among gay men helped to mobilize the gay community to fight HIV/AIDS. The gay rights movement also helped to increase the participation of gay men in HIV prevention programs. Two decades later, African Americans who are most at risk of infection are less willing to participate in an HIV prevention program than white gay men were during the initial years of the epidemic. Offering a program to African-American men on the down low or to African-American women who have not been reached by HIV prevention programs employing conventional strategies is onerous and often ineffective. Thus, a vital need arises for effective HIV prevention strategies that effectively attract these hard-to-reach populations.

One promising way to engage African Americans who are members of hidden populations is by using family-focused HIV prevention programs. Family-focused interventions have demonstrated considerable effectiveness in the reduction of drug and alcohol abuse as well as in tobacco use among youth (Brooks and Rice, 1997). Yet only in recent years have HIV researchers and practitioners begun to employ interventions focusing on the family. Many of these initiatives emerged as a result of a request for proposals that appeared in 1987 by the National Institute of Mental Health for family-focused

HIV prevention interventions. Family-focused HIV interventions share common characteristics that require consideration when designing ways to reach at-risk hidden African-American men and women. As shown in Table 6.1, these characteristics are grouped into five categories: (1) focal family member(s); (2) family member change agent(s); (3) intervention technology; (4) intervention deliverer; and (5) intervention setting.

Describing each briefly, the *focal family member* is the individual or members in the family for whom the intervention is designed to prevent or reduce their risk behavior. For example, the family-focused intervention Keepin' It R.E.A.L.! was developed to postpone sexual intercourse among adolescents (ages eleven to fourteen). This intervention focused on youths and their mothers with a curriculum designed to increase the mothers' confidence in discussing sexual health issues with their adolescents, to increase the adolescents' confidence in resisting pressures to initiate sexual intercourse before they are ready, and to enhance their confidence to use safer-sex practices when they do become sexually active (Diorio et al., 2000). Similarly, Krauss and colleagues' (2000) Parent/Preadolescent Training for HIV Prevention (PATH) program was designed to help parents be effective HIV educators for their children.

Perhaps not surprisingly, similar to the family-focused interventions designed to reduce drug use among youths, many family-focused HIV prevention programs center on reducing risky behaviors among youths. A number of family-focused HIV prevention programs have begun to focus on adults. The structural ecosystems therapy (SET) program developed by Mitrani, Szapocznik, and Batista serves as an example of one of these programs (Mitrani, Szapocznik, and Batista, 2000). SET focuses on adult African-American women who are HIV positive. Since the emphasis is on the family, not on the individual, members of at-risk groups are more inclined to participate in the program.

Family change agent refers to the individual in the family through whom the intervention effects are moderated. In using family-focused interventions, HIV prevention practitioners and researchers should take caution not to confuse the role of the family member as a change agent with that of the focal family member thus misdirecting a program intended to prevent the risk behavior of a mother by focusing on other adults in the family. Members of hidden populations are often

TABLE 6.1. Common Domains of Family-Focused Interventions

Focal Family Member(s)	Family Change Agent	Intervention Technology	Technology Delivering Agent	Setting
Child	Mother	Parenting skills building	Professionals, peers	Community, home
Child's parents, siblings	Child	Assertiveness and problem-solving skills building	Community members, professionals, peers	School, community
Woman's parents, siblings, spouse, and children	HIV-positive woman	Psychosocial skills building, networking skills building	Professionals, HIV-positive peers	Community

more inclined to become involved in a program when they become the family change agent rather than the target.

Intervention technology is used to refer to methods employed to bring about a change in behavior. HIV prevention specialists have long recognized that knowledge combined with skill-building activities are necessary to effectively bring about a behavior change. Technology is an equally important factor to consider in designing ways to involve members of a hidden population. Many adults are not inclined to participate in a program that lacks interactive and stimulating experiences. To insure that participants remain in the program, the intervention technology must be tailored to their needs and interests. For example, for women, an emphasis on learning better ways to promote the health and success of their children and themselves may induce them to participate. For African-American men, use of technologies that focus on improving relationships with one's child serve as an incentive to participate. For men who are experiencing severe financial stress, such as men who have recently been released from prison, combining an HIV prevention program with a job-seeking program may function as a strong inducement to participate in a program.

Just as the intervention technology is important, so too is the *intervention deliverer*. The term intervention deliverer is used to refer to individuals such as professional facilitators, peer facilitators, or community members, who are responsible to deliver the intervention technology to the family change agents and the focal family member. Getting a member of a hidden population to participate in an HIV prevention program is only half the battle. Some studies with youths, however, have revealed peers to be as effective as professionals in delivering an intervention (Jemmott, Jemmott, and Fang, 1998). Parent peers are more effective than professionals in delivering an intervention to lower-income, less-educated, African-American parents (Icard, 2001).

Last is the importance of the *intervention setting* for involving at-risk hidden populations in HIV prevention programs. Family-focused interventions can be delivered in the home, school, or community depending on the nature of the interventions and the needs of the family change agents and focal family members. The concern here is to provide the intervention in an environment that offers a feeling of safety from the scrutiny of the general public and the African-American community. Providing an HIV prevention program in a community center, employment office, or similar site that tends to be non-health related is preferable to offering programs in traditional health settings.

FACTORS TO CONSIDER

Political, financial, and social barriers often block HIV prevention and treatment programs from reaching those who are at highest risk of infection such as African Americans (CDC, 2001a). Several factors require consideration in developing effective strategies for reaching hard-to-reach populations. Included among those factors are:

1. *Correctly identifying and targeting hidden populations:* Hard-to-reach or hidden populations can be identified by age, gender, education, income status, race, and ethnicity. Among African Americans, African-American young and adult MSM, African-American women (especially women with lower income and limited education), and African-American adolescents (particularly youths from families experiencing chronic economic stress) are most vulnerable to HIV infection and comprise the hidden populations that should be targeted by family-based interventions. The use of family-focused interventions to involve these subgroups in HIV prevention helps to decrease the stigma.

2. *Understanding the contextual features of the family:* The family composition in hidden or hard-to-reach populations is quite diverse and can include traditional two-parent families, single-parent families, stepfamilies, and extended kin families. In many cases, families have nonbiological relationships as their functional core. In recognition of this fact, the National Institute of Mental Health (NIMH) Consortium on Family and HIV/AIDS defined *family* as a network of mutual commitments. These commitments are characterized by perceived strength and duration of relationships, perceived financial, emotional, and instrumental support, as well as perceived conflict (Pequegnat and Szapocznik, 2000). Thus, persons who fulfill relationship roles traditionally specified by biological and legal relationships are considered family members for the purpose of HIV/AIDS prevention (Mellins et al., 1996). In their analysis of families with

AIDS, Pequegnat and Szapocznik (2000) suggest that service providers construct a genogram with their clients to more effectively identify family networks. A similar procedure called eco-mapping may be useful for the identification of individuals who may have influence on the HIV risk behavior of individuals being targeted through family-based HIV prevention programs. The difference between these two technologies is worth noting. Ecomaps, which apply the biological concept of ecosystems to human communities, are flow diagrams that portray the interrelationship of family and community systems over time (Hartman, 1979). Genograms, on the other hand, focus primarily on biological family relationships, and hence, would be less useful in successfully defining kinship networks for family-focused interventions directed toward hidden at-risk African Americans.

3. *Selecting an appropriate, nonstigmatized name:* The name of the family-focused intervention project plays an important role in conveying the message, nature, and focus of the project to the community. The name of the project should reflect the key principles of the program one wishes to emphasize, that is, the strengths and positive aspects of the program and/or the aspects of the family on which the project focuses. For example, a family-focused intervention project centered on parent-child relationships that is currently being implemented is Teaming African-American Parents for Survival Skills (TAAPSS). Avoid using the terms HIV and AIDS in the name or title of the project because the stigma attached to HIV/AIDS may deter the target population from participating in the project.

CONCLUSION

Lower levels of education and income, limiting cultural values and attitudes, and involvement in stigmatized or illegal activities, such as drug use and prostitution, contribute to at-risk African Americans being elusive or difficult to involve as participants in HIV prevention programs. These hidden populations present unique challenges to HIV prevention practitioners and researchers. One viable alternative for HIV prevention practitioners and researchers to consider for successfully involving at-risk hidden segments of the African-American population is family-focused interventions.

As such, family-based interventions offer HIV prevention practitioners and researchers several advantages over other conventionally focused interventions. One advantage these programs offer is that, by focusing on the family, less attention is directed to stigmatized groups such as MSM, victims of domestic violence, and substance abusers. Second, family-focused intervention has the potential to provide a more comprehensive or holistic approach to HIV prevention, e.g., designing a family-based intervention that integrates strengthening social support and sexual-risk-reduction efforts. Finally, inherent in the family-based intervention model is the sheer number of people that may be impacted. Family members not intentionally targeted for intervention still become more aware of HIV/AIDS infection and its relation to risky behaviors; they can also become mechanisms for information dissemination themselves.

Much remains unknown about family-based interventions. Practitioners and researchers alike remain unclear as to what type of intervention is most effective for engaging and changing risk behaviors of particular hidden populations. Likewise, very little is known about the effectiveness of family-based interventions for various family configurations including fathers and sons and same-sex couples. Further attention is required both to the science and technology of family-based HIV interventions. This includes such areas as parent-child communication, parental modeling, communication dynamics and processes between adult family members, and length of and times for delivering interventions. Notwithstanding these concerns, the use of family-focused interventions as a means of approaching hidden populations is promising.

REFERENCES

AIDS Action (2001). Incarcerated populations and HIV/AIDS. *Policy Facts.* Washington, DC: Author.

Alexander, J.F, Robbins, M.S., and Sexton, T.L. (2000). Family-based interventions with older, at-risk youth: From promise to proof to practice. *Journal of Primary Prevention, 21*(2), 185-205.

Brooks, C.S. and Rice, K.F. (1997). *Families in recovery: Coming full circle.* Baltimore, MD: Paul H. Brookes Publishing Co.

Bull, J. (2001). PA imprisons blacks at highest rate. *Post-Gazette,* July 29.

Centers for Disease Control and Prevention (1990). Risk behaviors for HIV transmission among intravenous-drug users not in drug treatment—United States, 1987-1989. *Mortality and Morbidity Weekly Report (MMWR), 39,* 273-276.

Centers for Disease Control and Prevention (1993). Assessment of street outreach for HIV prevention—selected sites, 1991-1993. *MMWR, 42,* 873, 879-880.

Centers for Disease Control and Prevention (1998). *HIV/AIDS Surveillance Report, 10*(2), 17.

Centers for Disease Control and Prevention (2000a). *HIV/AIDS Surveillance Report, 12*(2), 1-44.

Centers for Disease Control and Prevention (2000b). *HIV/AIDS Surveillance Report, 12*(1).

Centers for Disease Control and Prevention (2001a). *HIV Prevention Strategic Plan through 2005.* Atlanta, GA: Author

Centers for Disease Control and Prevention (2001b). State-specific pregnancy and birth rates among teenagers—United States, 1991-1992. *MMWR, 50*(21), 430-434.

Cummings, G.L., Battle, R., Barker, J., and Krasnovsky, F. (1997). HIV risk among low-income African-American mothers of elementary school children. *Journal of Health and Social Policy, 8*(3), 27-39.

Diaz, R.D., Ayala, G., and Bein, E. (1999). Social oppression, resiliency and sexual risk: Findings from the national Latino gay men's study. Presented at the National HIV Prevention Conference, Atlanta, Georgia, August 29-September 1. Abstract #287.

Dilorio, C., Resnicow, K., Denzmore, P., Rogers-Tillman, G., Wang, D.T., Dudley, W.N., Lipana, J., and Van Marter, D.F. (2000). Keepin' It R.E.A.L! A mother-adolescent HIV prevention program. In W. Pequegnat and J. Szapocznik (Eds.), *Working with families in the era of HIV/AIDS* (pp. 113-132). Thousand Oaks, CA: Sage.

El-Bassel, N., Gilbert, L., Krishnan, S., Gaeta, T., Schilling, R.F., and Witte, S. (1999). Partner abuse and sexual risk behavior among women receiving care from emergency departments. *Violence and Victims, 13*(4), 1-17.

El-Bassel, N., Gilbert, L., Rajah, V., Foleno, A., and Frye, V. (2000). Fear and violence: Raising the HIV stakes. *AIDS Education and Prevention, 12*(2), 154-170.

El-Bassel, N., Gilbert, L., Rajah, V., Foleno, A., and Frye, V. (2001). Social support among women in methadone treatment who experience partner violence: Isolation and male controlling behavior. *Violence Against Women, 7*(3), 246-274.

Gary, L. E. (1978). *Mental health: A challenge to the black community.* Philadelphia, PA: Dorrance.

Gray, M. and Littlefield, M. B. (2002). Black women and addictions. In S. L. A. Straussner and S. Brown (Eds.), *The handbook of addiction treatment for women: Theory and practice* (pp. 301-322). San Francisco: Jossey-Bass.

Hartman, A. (1979). *Finding families: An ecological approach to family assessment in adoption.* Thousand Oaks, CA: Sage.

Icard, L. (2002). Empowering families to reduce HIV. NIHM Conference on the Role of Families in Preventing and Adapting to HIV/AIDS, July 24-26, Miami, FL.

Jemmott, J.B, Jemmott, L.S., and Fong, G.T. (1998). Abstinence and safer sex HIV risk-reduction interventions for African-American adolescents. *Journal of the American Medical Association, 279*(19), 1529-1536.

Krauss, B.J., Godfrey, C., Yee, D., Goldsamt, L., Tiffany, J., Almeyda, L., Davis, W.R., Bula, E., Reardon, D., Jones, Y., et al. (2000). Saving our children from a silent epidemic: The PATH program for parents and preadolescents. In W. Pequegnat and J. Szapocznik (Eds.), *Working with families in the era of HIV/AIDS* (pp. 89-112). Thousand Oaks, CA: Sage.

Malcolm, A., Aggleton, P., Bronfman, M., Galvao, J., Mane, P., and Verrall, J. (1998). HIV-related stigmatization and discrimination: Its forms and contexts. *Critical Public Health, 8*(4), 347-370.

Mellins, C.A., Ehrhardt, A.A., Newman, L., and Conard, M. (1996). Selective kin: Defining the caregivers and families of children with HIV disease. In A. O'Leary and L.S. Jemmott (Eds.), *Women and AIDS: Coping and care. AIDS prevention and mental health* (pp. 123-149). New York: Plenum Press.

Metzger, D.S., Woody, G.E, McLellan, A.T., O'Brien, C. P., Druley, P., Navaline, H., De Philippis, D., Stolley, P., and Abrutyn, E. (1993). Human immunodeficiency virus seroconversion among intravenous drug users in and out of treatment: An 18-month prospective follow-up. *Journal of Acquired Immune Deficiency Syndrome, 6*,1049-1056.

Mitrani, V.B, Szapocznik, J., and Batista, C.R. (2000). Structural ecosystems therapy with HIV+ African-American women. In W. Pequegnat and J. Szapocznik (Eds.), *Working with families in the era of HIV/AIDS* (pp. 243-279). Thousand Oaks, CA: Sage.

Pequegnat, W. and Szapocznik, J. (2000). *Working with families in the era of HIV/AIDS.* Thousand Oaks, CA: Sage.

Siegal, H.A., Carlson, R.G., Falck, R., Li, L., Forney, M. A., Rapp, R. C., Baumgartner, K., Myers, W., and Nelson, M. (1991). HIV infection and risk behaviors among intravenous drug users in low seroprevalence areas in the Midwest. *American Journal Public Health, 81,* 1642-1644.

Stewart, D.L., Zuckerman, C.L., and Inge, J.M. (1994). HIV seroprevalence in a chronically mentally ill population. *Journal of the National Medical Association, 86,* 519-523.

Stokes, J.P. and Peterson, J.L. (1998). Homophobia, self-esteem, and risk for HIV among African-American men who have sex with men. *AIDS Education and Prevention, 10*(3), 278-292.

U.S. Department of Justice (1999). *Update: HIV/AIDS, STDs and TB in correctional facilities.* Washington, DC: Author.

Valleroy, L.A., MacKellar, D.A., Karon, J.M., Janssen, R.S., and Hayman, C.R. (1998). HIV infection in disadvantaged out-of-school youth: Prevalence for U.S.

Jobs Corps entrants, 1990 through 1996. *Journal of Acquired Immune Deficiency Syndrome, 19,* 67-73.

Valleroy, L.A., MacKellar, D.A., Karon, J.M., Rosen, D.H., McFarland, W., Shehan, D.A., Stoyanoff, S.R., LaLota, M., Celentano, D.D., Koblin, B.A., et al. (2000). HIV prevalence and associated risks in young men who have sex with men. *Journal of the American Medical Association, 284*(2), 198-204.

Chapter 7

HIV/AIDS Among African Americans in the Mississippi/Louisiana Delta Region: A Macro-Practice Empowerment Model

Peggy Pittman-Munke
Vincent J. Venturini

STATEMENT OF THE PROBLEM

Rural areas face unique challenges with regard to HIV/AIDS, both in terms of prevention and treatment. These challenges are complicated by the fact that rural areas in general are more likely to condemn deviant behavior and are more likely to enforce social norms in order to maintain the current social order (Moses and Bruchner, 1980). This is especially true of rural, predominately African-American communities. One major obstacle to proactive work in both prevention and treatment is the fundamentalist religious value base and the belief system about homosexuality that characterizes many sectors of the African-American community as well as sectors of the dominant culture. The power of this value base is intensified in rural areas where there is a large African-American population and where the church is the dominant social institution. Nowhere in the United States is this more apparent than in the Delta region of Mississippi and Louisiana. Because of the comparatively high percentage of rural African Americans infected with HIV/AIDS, it is important to provide a model of practice which is culturally compatible with this population. However, the proposed model also can serve communities that are neither predominantly African American, nor predominantly rural, but which are conservative in religious and moral values. The model could also be adapted to work through social institutions other than the church.

The conservative political climate of rural Mississippi and rural Louisiana makes it difficult to deal proactively with HIV/AIDS, complicating both prevention and treatment. The Delta area of Louisiana and Mississippi, the focus of this chapter, is largely African American. The church is generally the center of the community. Churches have an emphasis on "traditional, moral" values. These values, grounded in fundamentalist religious belief, are slow to change (Rounds, 1988). Delta churches are largely fundamentalist, mostly Southern Baptist and Pentecostal. The teachings of these churches are generally homophobic in nature. In part, for this reason, Southern Baptist and Pentecostal denominations have not developed groups such as Integrity (Episcopal), Dignity (Roman Catholic), and Affirmation (United Methodist) which offer support to homosexual persons within the context of the church. Even if such support existed within the denomination on the national level, this would make little difference in the Delta region, where pastors generally pay scant allegiance to church structures beyond the local area. In general, most fundamentalist churches hold religious doctrines that view homosexuality as a sin, a crime, or a mental illness (Boswell, 1980). This is certainly true of most Delta churches. A further complication of the lives of those diagnosed with HIV/AIDS results because rural Americans, particularly African Americans, often rely on church-based support networks or kin networks rather than the secular, bureaucratic resources in the community, even if such are available. The belief system of many churches often cuts off rural African Americans who are HIV/AIDS positive from church-based support networks. This effectively leaves this group with no resources other than those they themselves can provide.

Local Norms and Religious Values

The characteristic culture of rural areas, which is made up of strict norms, typically is not hospitable to people who deviate from these norms. Persons who are gay or lesbian and persons who are diagnosed with HIV/AIDS are viewed as deviating from traditional norms. In many rural areas, the Bible is the primary guide for behavior as well as the source of moral ideas. Local rural churches in the Delta region hold fast to biblical prohibitions against "being homosexual." Therefore, being gay is seen as "living outside the will of God" (Smith,

1997, p. 16). Community strictures resulting from this viewpoint make HIV/AIDS prevention efforts nearly impossible in many rural areas.

Socioeconomic Characteristics of the Delta Region

The Mississippi portion of the Delta is tellingly described by *Clarion-Ledger* staff writer Butch John as "7,600 square miles and home to roughly 508,000 people" and "lies between hope and hopelessness—between dreams and chronic desperation, grand vision and numbing complacency" (John, 1999).

The Delta region has serious problems. It still suffers from a "plantation mentality," and is characterized by extremes of wealth and poverty (Fairclough, 1995). The Center for Community Development at Delta State University (n.d.) in Cleveland, Mississippi describes the Mississippi Delta as an area of "pervasive, chronic rural poverty and extensive economic underdevelopment." Mississippi and Louisiana each have forty-five counties characterized as Delta counties, that is, the majority of counties in both states.

Historically, the Mississippi Delta area has been so impoverished over a long period of time that its counties consistently ranked among the worst in the nation in most lists of social and health indicators. Conditions of poverty, illiteracy, and poor health are woven together so tightly that it is nearly impossible to disentangle the strands (Rossilli, 1999). Recent statistics show this clearly. Fifteen Delta counties in Mississippi had higher unemployment rates than the state's 5.5 percent average in the 1998-1999 fiscal year, fourteen exceeded the state's average poverty level, and eight had double-digit unemployment. "In the 1990 census, the last time the comparison was made, 13 Delta counties ranked among America's 80 poorest counties nationally" (John, 1999). Furthermore, fifteen Delta counties exceed the state average for welfare and food stamp payments. More than half of the Mississippi Delta's counties have double the Mississippi average in these categories (John, 1999).

Census figures show that fewer than half of the residents of eight Mississippi counties have a high school education (John, 1999). In Madison Parish (County) Louisiana, 53 percent of the residents twenty-five years or older lack a high school diploma. Low educational attainment also complicates HIV/AIDS prevention (Rural Empowerment Zone and Enterprise Community Program, n.d.).

The fact that the Delta region is overwhelmingly rural also poses significant problems. There are a few population centers amid decaying communities and a few large plantations and a "growing, aging, underclass for whom services such as welfare payments are no longer available" (John, 1999). Jackson State University economics professor Dal Didia locates the Delta among the United States's most economically deprived areas, rivaling South Central Los Angeles and inner cities of Detroit and Chicago (John, 1999). Others compare the Delta to a developing country.

Other problems include the high rate of out-of-wedlock births. Nine Delta counties are among the ten Mississippi counties with the highest percentage of out-of-wedlock births. Five Delta counties rank among the state's worst for infant mortality (Rossilli, 1999). A related issue is the lack of accessibility to health care, although for many Delta residents, health care is lower on their list of priorities than "more important necessities such as food, housing and water supply." Each of the Delta counties is considered by the federal government to be a medically underserved area (Rossilli, 1999). Heart disease and diabetes are major problems. Health issues are complicated by the fact that "to many, illness is an unexplained phenomena, not something science based" and as a result "children grow up with no understanding of what causes illness or how to prevent it" (Rossilli, 1999). This fact also greatly complicates HIV/AIDS prevention and treatment.

AFRICAN AMERICANS AND THE RISK OF HIV/AIDS

African Americans are at particular risk for HIV/AIDS. "While African Americans comprise 13% of the U.S. population, they are disproportionately affected by HIV, accounting for 37% of total AIDS cases in the United States" according to 1998 statistics reported by the Centers for Disease Control (CDC) (University of California at San Francisco, 1999). In 2002, 42,746 AIDS cases were recorded by the CDC. Of those cases, 14,310 were reported among African-American males over the age of thirteen, and 7,339 cases were reported among African-American women over the age of thirteen (CDC, 2003). Often, women do not realize that they are infected until they give birth to an infected child.

In the Delta region, poverty plays a major role in lack of access to adequate medical care. Injection-drug-related AIDS is a major issue in the region. Through the end of 1996, 610 Mississippi residents ages thirteen and older had injection-drug-related AIDS or had died of it. About 20 percent of all AIDS cases in Mississippi are drug-injection related. Through the end of 1996, some 376 African Americans living in Mississippi had injection-drug-related AIDS or had died from it. The rate of injection-drug-related AIDS cases among blacks in Mississippi is four times higher than the rate for whites (Dogwood Center, n.d.). Nationally, African Americans also account for over half (53 percent) of all AIDS cases among injection drug users. It is a harsh truth that 62 percent of all children with AIDS are African American (University of California at San Francisco, 1999). The infection of children with HIV makes it crucial that even conservative, largely African-American rural regions, deal effectively with the issues of HIV/AIDS prevention and treatment. Sexual behavior also must be addressed, because the major cause of HIV/AIDS among African-American men is sexual activity with infected partners. Unfortunately, because of the cultural prohibitions against homosexual activity, many men continue to have unprotected sex with women, who then become infected. The CDC points out that among African-American men, the cumulative proportion of AIDS cases attributed to homosexual or bisexual activity (38 percent) is greater than that attributed to injection drug use (35 percent) (CDC, 1998). Finding a way to reach this population is critical. However, as high as these rates seem, rates of HIV/AIDS in rural areas do not include the persons incarcerated in federal prisons, which are often located in rural areas (Mancoske, 1997). The figures include only people living in the region who are not incarcerated. This chapter does not include material related to practice with prison populations.

HIV/AIDS IN RURAL AMERICA

The growth of aids in rural America is a major concern to the Centers for Disease Control and Prevention (CDC). AIDS is growing rapidly among rural Americans. Rural HIV/AIDS case rates more than doubled from 4.9 per 100,000 people in 1991 to 10.1 in 1996. Although rural case rates are still lower than city rates, city rates have been dropping while rural rates have been rising (Van Sant, 1998).

AIDS in rural areas tends to be largely a minority issue, affecting both men and women. Often AIDS is spread through heterosexual contact. This holds true in the Delta counties of Louisiana and Mississippi. Feinlieb and Michael (1998) point out that the number of rural adults who have reduced risky sexual behavior is small compared to urban/suburban adults. Widespread denial of vulnerability to HIV infection is common among rural residents, in part because of the prevailing religious climate.

Although attitudes in the African-American community are changing slowly, homophobia and negative attitudes toward gay males are still prevalent. The impact of these attitudes is serious, and this, along with a lack of understanding of disease, prevents many from taking adequate precautions. Some of the results of these negative stereotypes for young homosexual African-American men are "low self-esteem, lack of community, and psychological distress, all of which contribute to risk taking behaviors" (Stokes and Peterson, 1998, p. 288). An examination of the effects of stereotypes on young African-American males is critical because one in four of all new HIV infections is estimated to occur in young people between the ages of thirteen and twenty.

Youth and HIV/AIDS: An American Agenda (White House Office of AIDS National Policy, 1996) presents a series of actions that can be taken to reduce the impact of HIV/AIDS on this population. The report makes clear that adolescents can protect themselves from HIV if they are given appropriate information and then helped to develop the skills to use the information. Suggested prevention strategies include the following:

- Parents can be the best teachers for their children.
- Sexual abstinence should be encouraged.
- HIV prevention should not be separated from STD prevention, pregnancy prevention, substance abuse prevention, sexuality education, self-esteem activities, and human development education.
- Successful prevention activities focus on providing access to accurate information and personalizing this information to moti-

vate change and provide training in behavioral skills to build competence, communication, and self-esteem.

- Sexuality education, when done properly, reflects the needs of the community and acknowledges the value of both abstinence and safer sex as tools to prevent HIV infection. (Rural Center for AIDS/STD Prevention, 1996).

However, most of these prevention activities are in conflict with prevailing cultural norms in the rural Delta region. Prevention is challenging in areas where cultural norms make it difficult to talk openly about HIV/AIDS and STD, and where there is little understanding of the causes of disease. Also, few resources are available to devote to prevention activities.

Barriers to prevention activities for youths in rural areas are greater than those in urban areas. The barriers include:

- limited resources available to youth-serving agencies (and limited resources in terms of agencies which serve youth);
- conservative and judgmental attitudes about sexuality education;
- lack of confidentiality in small communities;
- hostility toward agency staff attempting to provide education/ services;
- youth boredom and isolation which leads to adolescent risk taking; and
- ignorance and denial among adolescents about personal risk for HIV infection (National Advocates for Youth, 1996).

These barriers loom large in the Delta region. Some proposed solutions to these issues include:

- development of intra-agency, interagency, and media support for HIV prevention programs;
- development of materials and programs relevant for rural youths: incorporating HIV education into existing youth health programs, involving youths, adapting existing resources, and creating materials which are age- and culturally appropriate; and
- creating alternatives to risky behavior (National Advocates for Youth 1996).

However, most of these solutions are either culturally insensitive to the Delta region, or ignore the reality of the limitations of already overstretched available resources.

PROPOSED PRACTICE MODEL FOR CULTURALLY SENSITIVE PRACTICE WITH AFRICAN AMERICANS

Other authors in this book have proposed practice models suitable for micro- and mezzo-level practice with people suffering from HIV/AIDS. The model proposed in this chapter will focus on macro practice in a rural region as well as on cultural sensitivity to the norms of rural African Americans.

The proposed model is focused on one of the major institutions of society, especially powerful in the Delta region, the African-American church. This proposed model relies on community in two senses, the rural community of place and the larger African-American religious community. Hixson (1998, p. 10) points out that a pattern of "piecemeal responses to individual problems has resulted in overly fragmented, specialized, and standardized assortment of services, programs, and policies." He reminds us that that this has been especially true in addressing the issues of substance abuse and "other health-related, socially destructive behaviors affecting African Americans" (Hixson, 1998, p. 10). Hixson (1998) raises another critical issue, the importance of exploring new possibilities for service delivery that are "deeply embedded in, build on, and leverage traditional cultural foundations and community strengths and resources" (p. 12). The proposed model fits within Hixson's construct.

"For most African Americans today, religion, often connected to church going, and spirituality are major sources for preventing, healing, and treating problems large or small" (Brisbane, 1998, p. 3). Although previously the Church has not been a focus for macro practice, Brisbane offers social workers an important resource to help move beyond traditional models of practice. The political climate of the first decade of the twenty-first century makes this movement not only feasible but also critical and timely in terms of securing needed resources. In the case of the rural Delta region of Louisiana and Mississippi, the emphasis on faith-based service delivery, as Brisbane (1998) points out, is a good cultural fit with the region. Social workers must join with pastors and church members to develop methods of dealing with both prevention and treatment of HIV/AIDS that fit within the culture of the region. In the funding climate of the George W. Bush administration, working with the faith-based community opens important avenues to receiving funds to support this work.

However, there are other reasons besides the need for funding to join with churches in order to effectively serve HIV/AIDS-infected African Americans. These reasons are related to community empowerment and community development. There is a need to go beyond the professional community and the constraints of outside funding to develop a model of practice with the HIV/AIDS population that will work successfully in this region. The empowerment model helps us to understand the strengths that lie within a given community. The HIV/AIDS community in the Delta region has many strengths which are often ignored by service providers. Park (1983) identifies essential characteristics of community: "The essential characteristics of a community . . . are those of (1) a population, territorially organized, (2) more or less completely rooted in the soil it occupies, (3) its individual units living in a relationship of mutual interdependence" (Park, 1983, p. 29). Utilization of Park's characteristics provides a guide to the construction of a useful model for practice based on an empowerment and a strengths perspective.

Kretzmann and McKnight (1993) explain that most communities often have unrecognized and unused assets. Saleebey (1997, p. 205) points out that "this is especially true of marginalized communities where individuals and groups have had to learn to survive under difficult and often rapidly changing conditions." Saleeby's statement describes the Delta region. An assets-based approach ensures that community assets should be utilized as a means of "working with and within a community" (p. 205). These assets are not just individual assets or assets of professional services within the community, but also those of natural helping networks and informal organizations in which the members of the HIV/AIDS community, including family members and friends, come together to both solve problems and to support one another. This clearly describes the church community in the Delta region.

The practice model proposed in this chapter is both assets and strengths based (Saleebey, 1997). The model seeks out the resources instead of focusing on the problems. The model is internally focused, so rather than emphasizing external factors and institutions, it examines the capacities and resources available within the group. The model is relationship driven with community as its essence. The worker thus begins with a capacity or strengths inventory, focused on area churches. The basic idea that supports this model is the connection of people with capacities to other people, associations, and institutions and to economic and other resources in the church.

In an assets-based model, services must be provided that consider cultural and social barriers. In an area as conservative as the Delta, services that focus strictly on disease and sexual orientation will alienate the community they propose to serve. Services delivered in this manner also ignore the increasing number of heterosexual women and men who are becoming infected. This group would not respond well to services and programs targeting homosexual behavior.

The affirmation of marginalized communities is critical. This means dealing with African-American youth, one of the fastest growing segments of the AIDS community. It also means acknowledging that HIV/AIDS is not limited to poor African Americans. Working-class and middle-class African Americans are also at risk. The culture of silence and shame connected to homosexuality fosters HIV transmission and increases risk not only for African-American men, but African-American women and children.

In planning HIV/AIDS prevention and treatment services in the Delta counties, it is clear that the organizations that must be targeted to provide the services are the churches. Because these counties of Louisiana and Mississippi are largely African American in their population, because the HIV/AIDS statistics also reflect a population that is also largely African American, and because in these rural counties the church is generally the center of the community, it is clear that the organizations that would be most effective with this population are the rural churches. Outsiders cannot provide prevention, education, or treatment in a way that will be well received by this population. Instead, these activities must take place within the churches. Those best able to mobilize this major resource are the pastors, elders, and the members. Since African-American churches are a powerful political base, the church can also provide a strong foundation from which to lobby for needed policies and funding and apply for dollars for services that are more available now to the faith-based community.

Balm in Gilead Model

Smith (1997) points out that rather than relying on social workers "to search out and find supports for gay people" suffering from HIV/AIDS in small rural communities, social workers need to ally with this population to develop a model for community practice based on organization and social action (Smith, 1997, pp. 16-17). African-American churches in the Delta, regardless of denomination, offer such an opportunity for community practice based on the model proposed by an organization called Balm in Gilead. Balm in Gilead works to prevent the further transmission of HIV among African peoples by mobilizing the religious community to address HIV appropriately and effectively (Seele, 2004a).

The Balm in Gilead model also fits well with the locality development model proposed by Rothman (1983). Locality development involves "the broad participation of a wide spectrum of people at the local community level in goal determination and action" (p. 25). In other words, community people determine their own needs and solve their own problems (Rothman, 1983, p. 25).

Seele (2004a) draws parallels with biblical times as she describes the model. In Gilead, a land ravaged by poor health care and racial discrimination among other ills, people suffered because of a lack of information and an inability to organize themselves to take political action. The ancient land of Gilead was similar in many ways to the modern Delta region of Louisiana and Mississippi and the way the HIV/AIDS epidemic is viewed.

The model of involvement proposed by Balm in Gilead is one that could be used by other African-American churches in the Delta region and elsewhere. The model is holistic, and it depends on total community involvement. However, a political action component and the incorporation of input by community members affected by HIV/AIDS would strengthen the model. The founder of the movement, Pernessa Seele, reflects on the history of African Americans in the United States when she calls on black churches to

> build upon the spiritual consciousness of our ancestors who were bound in the shackles of slavery. In pain and sorrow, they reached into the scriptures and wrote a song that bears witness to God's omnipotent and omnipresent nature that heals, forgives and loves unconditionally.

She continues with the history of African-American survival in the United States when she points out:

> Our ancestors . . . gave instructions to go, teach and to take responsibility for each other. The balm . . . enables us to fearlessly fight AIDS—whether on the front line of political action and HIV/AIDS education . . . or in the mine fields of a person's discriminatory thoughts against those infected and affected by HIV/AIDS. (Seele, 2004a)

Seele points out that combating HIV requires "bold, steadfast leadership." She reminds us that only the institutional church can effectively mobilize the black community and provide information that will be considered acceptable and credible. Seele views the African-American church as the logical source of prevention education and of support for individuals "infected and affected by HIV/AIDS" because it is still respected by the African-American community. Passionately, she avows that "only when churches are willing to admit that people living with AIDS are not 'them'; only when our churches recognize that AIDS is not . . . confined to those outside the faith community, can we begin to be effective" (Seele, 2004b).

Seele makes telling points that apply to the Delta region. She explains that orphaned children and teenagers who contract HIV/AIDS through ignorance and die before reaching their twenty-fifth birthdays, as well as abused mothers who are forced into unprotected sex with their infected husbands, are the innocent casualties of AIDS. She explains that there is still neither a vaccine nor a cure for this disease. She questions if there is a solution—"a balm in Gilead"—and answers her own question by reminding the reader that the church can be the balm if it will "take the appropriate steps to organize, mobilize, educate, and reach out" (Seele, 2004b).

Seele reminds us of the importance of this issue to African Americans and African-American churches by providing the statistics of AIDS incidence in the United States: three-fourths of all women who are HIV positive are African American, and more than four-fifths of all children infected with HIV are African American. She adds to these chilling statistics the fact that African-American teens have an infection rate that doubles every year. She concludes, "Wherever AIDS is present . . . statistics reveal that Africans and those in the African diaspora are disproportionately affected by HIV/AIDS" (Seele, 2004a).

Practitioners who are church members can bring the model to the attention of their pastors by sharing information about Balm in Gilead. The fact that it was developed by a national African-American church-based organization should make pastors more likely to embrace the model. Because the information on HIV/AIDS and the facts about HIV/AIDS and African Americans are directed toward pastors through a religious resource rather than coming through secular sources, practitioners are more likely to enlist their pastors to spearhead the effort to educate church members, as they learn the facts about HIV/AIDS. In addition, Balm in Gilead has the resources to provide pastors with factual data about the national support of clergy, pastors, congregation, and national denominational leaders for this effort in a culturally appropriate context. Practitioners could suggest that these resources, under the direction of the pastors, could also be used by community agencies to plan culturally appropriate interventions.

The national center for Balm in Gilead supplies easily adaptable ideas for use on the local level, including:

- Joining with other African-American churches in The Black Church Week of Prayer for the Healing of AIDS which is sponsored nationally by the Balm in Gilead.
- Hosting a prayer vigil for people with HIV/AIDS and their family members during The Black Church Week of Prayer for the Healing of AIDS. The Black Church Week of Prayer for the Healing of AIDS is an awareness program designed to educate and mobilize African-American religious congregations to become community centers of HIV prevention, treatment education, and compassionate care. The Week of Prayer begins each year on the first Sunday in March.
- Hosting an educational conference through the local ministers' association or through individual churches, depending on the needs of the area. Practitioners could be invited to add a health fair component to the conference.
- Distributing HIV/AIDS information at the churches.
- Talking with the men, women, youth, children, elderly, married couples, and single persons in the congregation about HIV/

AIDS as a part of the Adult Education ministry of the church. The organization offers spiritually based, culturally relevant books, articles, and videos to help with these discussions if needed.

These videos, books, and articles could be used in communitywide education as well.

The Balm in Gilead suggests beginning ministries within the church to deal with the needs of those suffering from HIV/AIDS. This fits with the way African-American churches historically have met physical and educational needs of their congregations as well as the spiritual needs. Although the model does not specifically state that those suffering from HIV/AIDS and their support systems should be involved in the development of ministries to deal with their needs, this is an important corollary to the success of the ministries. An addition to the model could be an invitation by the churches to local agencies to participate in carrying out many of these ministries. Ministries could include such activities as:

- Establishing care teams to assist people with HIV/AIDS and their family members at home.
- Spending time with the ill person, so that family members can have a break.
- Providing transportation for persons with HIV/AIDS to medical facilities.
- Including people with HIV/AIDS and their family members in church food and clothing ministries.
- Adding people with HIV/AIDS and their family members to church visitation lists.
- Praying for people with HIV/AIDS and their family members regularly.
- Filling out forms for the ill person, so that needed services can be obtained.
- Providing linkage to local and regional service providers.

The national organization also provides direct assistance to churches through the provision of training, education, resource materials, and guidance as well as by assisting in the planning, implementation, and evaluation of local HIV/AIDS activities, such as educational workshops or community care teams, and by suggesting regional speakers and organizations with which to collaborate.

The Balm in Gilead organization goes beyond palliative and prevention measures. It provides ongoing technical assistance to support HIV education and prevention activities within African-American churches and to assist collaborations between African-American faith organizations and state and local departments of health, medical, and social service providers and community-based organizations. It also operates the nation's only HIV/AIDS technical assistance center designed specifically to serve African American churches as well as public agencies and community-based organizations that wish to work with African-American churches on AIDS issues. This sort of backup support is critical for churches that lack access to sophisticated resources, such as those in rural regions like the Delta region of Mississippi and Louisiana. (To obtain technical assistance, send an e-mail to <info@balmingilead.org> or call the center at 1-888-225-6243.)

The primary purposes of the technical assistance center are:

- to increase the ability of African-American churches to access and use current, theoretically grounded knowledge about behavioral and social interventions for preventing HIV transmission;
- to provide support to infected and affected persons; and
- to access funding and other resources available for HIV education and prevention activities.

The secondary purpose of the center is to increase the cultural competence of public health professionals and other medical and direct service providers to work appropriately and effectively with the African-American faith community. The center's resources empower African-American churches to develop useful information for political lobbying and to access funding. Through the use of the center's resources, individual African-American churches can educate professionals throughout the region to serve those suffering with HIV/AIDS in a manner compatible with the moral base of the region.

The use of the center's resources adds legitimacy to efforts to attract resources and outside funding to the Delta region. The center maintains five panels of experts with national reputations who ensure that the center's services are grounded in scientific research, informed by the latest theories, and are appropriate for use by the target audiences. All of the activities of the center are evaluated by Columbia University's School of Public Health. All resource materials and education protocols that have been developed by the center are for use by African-American churches and public health professionals and are also reviewed by the School of Public Health.

Homan (1999) presented a number of elements that are useful in infusing change into a community. These elements correlate closely to the model sponsored by Balm in Gilead. The elements include (pp. 37-38).

- *Building on community assets.* The Balm in Gilead does this through utilizing the strengths of African-American church structures and the individual strengths of the members.
- *Increasing the skills of individuals.* The Balm in Gilead provides information and technical assistance, which increases the skills of both pastors and church members.
- *Connecting existing resources.* The Balm in Gilead not only encourages churches to connect with other community resources but also provides technical assistance to help with this.
- *Creating or increasing community resources.* The Balm in Gilead focuses on creating programs and resources through the churches, and through church linkage with various community organizations.
- *Encouraging the community to assume ownership of direction, action, and resources.* The Balm in Gilead has designed its model so that the individual churches determine the direction of the interventions, lead the action, and develop resources using the resources of the national organization as a basis for modification to fit the needs of the local churches.
- *Promoting the expectation that the community members will do all work possible.* The model encourages church members to take charge of developing resources appropriate to the needs of the church and the community. The resources are expected to be morally and culturally compatible with the church and the region as well.

The Balm in Gilead model, using Homan's (1999) elements as a guide, supports the infusion of change into Delta communities in a way that fits the values of the region. It is a model that expects leadership from within the African-American churches, which are the outward manifestations of the morals and values of the region. The model builds on assets already present, but is designed to encourage the development of additional human and resource assets within the community. The model begins with the churches, but soon incorporates all available community assets and resources. Change is infused into the community in a way that is culturally compatible and at a pace dictated by community desires and needs. The model deals with prevention activities as well as treatment services. An important part of the Balm in Gilead is that the prevention activities can be related to church values and local mores, while treatment services may deal only with the biblical injunction to care for the ill and infirm without judgment.

The Balm in Gilead model calls for infusing change into a community in a way that is both culturally relevant to the Mississippi Delta region and respectful of the most important institution in the Delta, the African-American church. The model is strengths based, both empowerment and assets based, and builds on both human and other resources already available in the region. Designed by African-American religious leaders for other African Americans, although it can be modified for use in other communities with other issues, this model has a better chance of success than secular models designed by the dominant culture. The model not only fits with the value base of the region but also is a good fit with the outlook of the Bush administration toward funding and services.

The Balm in Gilead model takes into account conservative religious norms and provides methods for both prevention and treatment of HIV/AIDS in a way that fits culturally with the Delta region. Because of the involvement of African-American pastors and the biblical basis of the model, the likelihood of acceptance by and use among church members is great. The concept of the churches as the initiators, with pastors and church members guiding social services and health care providers, is one which should be most appealing to powerful protectors of a traditional value base, both in the Mississippi Delta and elsewhere. The fact that the model was developed by an African-American religious leader for other African-American religious leaders should foster the acceptance of the model by the many who are rightfully skeptical of models of service that originate within the dominant culture.

The model proposed in this chapter is a generalist practice model, which, although a model of community-based practice, functions on all systems' levels. It calls for organizing within the churches and within the HIV/AIDS community, educating on an individual basis church members who are connected to the HIV/AIDS community, reminding pastors of the appropriate biblical injunctions to care for the site, setting up groups to minister within the church, and mobilizing the power of the African-American churches for community education, care of the sick, and political lobbying. This kind of assets-based community development model not only is empowering, but can be an important strategy to improve the physical and emotional quality of life for members of the HIV/AIDS community on the Mississippi Delta, while affirming their dignity and worth.

REFERENCES

Boswell, J. (1980). *Christianity, social tolerance, and homosexuality.* Chicago: University of Chicago Press.

Brisbane, F. (Ed.) (1998). *Cultural competence for health care professionals working with African-American communities: Theory and practice.* Washington, DC: DHHS.

Center for Community Development, Delta State University (n.d.). Background. Available online at: <http://www.deltast.edu/ccd/html_files/background.html>, accessed March 22, 2001.

Centers for Disease Control (1998). *HIV/AIDS Surveillance Report, 10,* 1-43.

Centers for Disease Control (2003). Acquired immunodeficiency syndrome (AIDS) cases, according to age at diagnosis, sex, detailed race, and Hispanic origin: United States, selected years 1985-2002. Available online at: <http://www.cdc.gov/nchs/data/hus/tables/2003/03hus053.pdf>, accessed February 17, 2004.

The Dogwood Center (n.d.). The epidemic of drug-related AIDS: Mississippi. Available online at: <http://drcnet.org/AIDS/ms_ban.html>, accessed February 17, 2004.

Fairclough, A. (1995). *Race and democracy: The civil rights struggle in Louisiana, 1915-1972.* Athens, GA: University of Georgia Press.

Feinlieb, J.A. and Michael, R.T. (1998). Reported changes in sexual behavior in response to AIDS in the United States. *Preventive Medicine, 27,* 400-411.

Hixson, J.D. (1998). Developing culturally anchored services: Confronting the challenge of intragroup diversity. In Brisbane, F. (Ed.), *Cultural competence for health care professionals working with African-American communities: Theory and practice* (pp. 9-46). Washington, DC: DHHS.

Homan, M.S. (1999). *Promoting community change: Making it happen in the real world.* Pacific Grove, CA: Brooks/Cole.

John, B. (1999). Incredible potential . . . incredible problems. *The Clarion-Ledger,* Internet edition, December 19. Available online at: <http://www.clarionledger. com/news/9912/19/19delta.html>, accessed March 22, 2001.

Kretzmann, J.P. and McKnight, J.L. (1993). *Building communities from the inside out.* Chicago: ACTA Publications.

Mancoske, R. (1997). Rural HIV/AIDS social services for gays and lesbians. In Smith, J.D. and Mancoske, R. (Eds.), *Rural gays and lesbians: Building on the strengths of communities* (pp. 37-52). Binghamton, NY: The Haworth Press.

Moses, A.E. and Bruchner, J.A. (1980). Special problems of rural gay clients. *Human Services in the Rural Environment, 5,* 22-27.

National Advocates for Youth (1996). *No immunity: Preventing HIV among rural youth.* Washington, DC: Author.

Park, R.E. (1983). Human ecology. In R.L. Warren and L. Lyon (Eds.), *New perspectives on the American community* (pp. 27-36). Homewood, IL: Dorsey Press.

Rossilli, M. (1999). Roots of ills in Delta—poverty. *The Clarion-Ledger,* Internet edition, December 22. Available online at: <http://www.clarionledger.com/ news/9912/ 22/19delta.html>, accessed March 22, 2001.

Rothman, J. (1983). Three models of community organization practice. In F. Cox, J. Erlich, J. Rothman, and J. Tropman (Eds.), *Strategies of community organization: A book of readings* (pp. 3-26). Itasca, IL: F.E. Peacock.

Rounds, K.A. (1988). AIDS in rural areas: Challenges to providing care. *Social Work, 33,* 257-261.

Rural Center for AIDS/STD Prevention (1996). *Rural Prevention Report, 3*(1/ Spring). Available online at: <http://www.indiana.edu/~aids/news/news5.html>, accessed February 17, 2004.

Rural Empowerment Zone and Enterprise Community Program (EZ/EC) (n.d.). Northeast Louisiana Delta Rural EC. Available online at: <http://www.ezec. gov/ezec/la/ladelta.html>, accessed September 15, 2000.

Saleebey, D. (1997). *The strengths perspective in social work practice.* New York: Longman.

Seele, P.C. (2004a). *AIDS, spirituality, and the African-American church: A call for a greater response.* Available online at: <http://www.balmingilead.org/resources/ spirituality.htm>, accessed February 17, 2004.

Seele, P.C. (2004b). The church's role in HIV prevention. Available online at: <http:// www.balmingilead.org/resources/churchrole.asp>, accessed February 17, 2004.

Smith, J.D. (1997). Working with larger systems: Rural lesbians and gays. In Smith, J.D. and Mancoske, R. (Eds.), *Rural gays and lesbians: Building on the strengths of communities* (pp. 13-21). Binghamton, NY: The Haworth Press.

Stokes, J.P. and Peterson, J.L. (1998). Homophobia, self esteem, and risk for HIV among African-American men who have sex with men. *AIDS Education and Prevention, 10,* 278-92.

University of California at San Francisco (1999). *What are African Americans' HIV Prevention Needs?* Available online at: <http://www.caps.scsf.edu/afamrev. html>, accessed April 9, 2000.

Van Sant, R. (1998). AIDS growing in rural region. *Cincinnati Post* (World Wide Web edition), July 13. Available online at: <http://www.cincypost.com/news/ 1998/hivrur071398.html>, accessed February 17, 2004.

White House Office of National AIDS Policy (1996). *Youth and HIV/AIDS: An American agenda.* Washington, DC: Author.

Chapter 8

Cultural Influences
on HIV/AIDS Prevention:
Louisiana African-American Women

Sybil G. Schroeder

INTRODUCTION

We have now experienced twenty years of HIV/AIDS infections in the United States. The total number of AIDS cases has increased each year from 1986 through 1995 and is now at pandemic levels. Although the number of cases among ethnic minorities began to decrease in 1994 (Centers for Disease Control and Prevention [CDC], 2000b), dramatic increases among African Americans have recently been reported in the number of cases of new HIV infections and cases of AIDS (CDC, 2000a,e).

During the late 1980s and early 1990s, educational information concerning HIV transmission and prevention became widespread in the United States. However, HIV/AIDS was often viewed by African Americans as primarily a gay white male disease, and secondary prevention through education focused on that group while sexually active heterosexuals remained at risk. Over time, community prevention education messages have targeted groups determined most at risk for HIV infection based upon statistical trends. However, even though women of color have become the focus of prevention programs, the numbers of new infections among this group continues to increase (Choi and Catania, 1996). In particular, African-American women in the South have become infected with HIV at even greater rates than in other parts of the United States. Since 1993, an increase has occurred in the proportion of HIV/AIDS cases among Louisiana females. In 1993, only 21 percent of AIDS cases in Louisiana were women. By 1999, 30 percent of all new infections were among women, 85 percent of which were African American (Louisiana Department of Health and Hospitals [LDHH], 2001c).

Although acknowledging a need for cultural sensitivity, HIV/AIDS prevention interventions classify African Americans as a homogenous group when historical, cultural, and regional differences should be considered. In her examination of AIDS and women of color, Land (1994) discussed women of color as a heterogeneous group of disenfranchised status, dispelling the myth of group homogeneity. Louisiana's women of color are descendants of slaves, free people of color, Creoles, and Cajuns, and from backgrounds from all parts of Africa, Europe, and the Caribbean. African-American women in Louisiana have a history of disenfranchisement, marginalization, and poverty unlike that of African-American women in other parts of the United States. According to the Institute for Women's Policy Research (IWPR, 1998), "Differences exist with respect to age, race, education, rural or urban residence, and other distinctions among women, and not all women enjoy equal access to Louisiana's political and economic resources" (p. 6). "The legacy of racism, coupled with cultural, religious, and sociopolitical factors, also influences the behavior of African-American women" (Land, 1994, p. 356).

The combination of culturally transmitted values and mores, and educational, professional, political, and health shortfalls makes African-American Louisiana women an ideal community for examining fundamental issues regarding the efficacy of HIV/AIDS prevention efforts. This chapter establishes a foundation for examination of this group by providing an overview of HIV/AIDS statistical data. It then addresses the ethnic and cultural landscape of Louisiana as a unique socialization vehicle from its historical foundations to its current manifestations. Finally, it explores the appropriateness of an ethnic epistemology coupled with a dual perspective or double-consciousness approach.

HIV/AIDS STATISTICAL OVERVIEW

The Centers for Disease Control and Prevention (CDC) is responsible for defining the epidemiological aspects of infectious diseases in the United States (Henderson, 1993). The CDC releases HIV/AIDS statistical data semiannually. HIV/AIDS have reached pandemic proportions since the early 1980s, and, in this country alone, affect approximately 1 million individuals (CDC, 2000a,e). The CDC (2000f) reports that currently 299,944 individuals live with an AIDS diagnosis and 113,167 are infected with HIV. James (1994) stated that for every case of AIDS, there are four cases of known HIV infection and eight to ten persons who are infected and unaware of their status.

African Americans make up approximately 12 percent of the population of the United States but are disproportionately represented among cases of HIV/AIDS. Statistics for 1997 reveal that African Americans represented 35.9 percent of all cases of AIDS (CDC, 1998). "In the first half of 1998, 15,556 cases of AIDS were reported among all minority racial/ethnic groups and accounted for 68 percent of all reported cases of AIDS in the United States" (CDC, 2000b, p. 1). By the end of 1998, the numbers among African Americans had cumulatively increased to 251,408, representing 36.5 percent of all AIDS cases (CDC, 1999a). Year-end statistics for 1999 reported that the number of AIDS cases among African Americans had increased to 272,881 or 37.2 percent of the cumulative number of cases (CDC, 2000a).

In 1998, the CDC began publishing data from thirty-three areas of the United States with confidential HIV infection reporting. These data show that the number of cases among African Americans far exceeds that of other racial groups. African Americans accounted for 55,953 cases of HIV infection by the end of 1998 (CDC, 1999b) and 64,299 by the end of 1999 (CDC, 2000e), representing 52.5 percent, and 52.4 percent, respectively.

Women are disproportionately impacted in the HIV/AIDS pandemic (Fields, 1992; National Pediatric HIV Resource Center, 1992; Satcher, 1994). In 1990, the CDC (1995) reported, "Prevention of HIV infection in women is critical for the control of the HIV epidemic in the United States and throughout the world" (p. 846). Fields (1992), the National Pediatric HIV Resource Center (1992), and Satcher (1994) subsequently reported that women represent the country's fastest growing population of newly diagnosed HIV and AIDS cases. By February 1993, the CDC reported that AIDS cases among women increased 17 percent between 1990 and 1991 and had become the sixth leading cause of death among U.S. women aged twenty-five to forty-four. Although in 1992 women accounted for

13.8 percent of persons living with AIDS (CDC, 1996), the proportion of women with AIDS had grown to 16 percent by the end of 1997 (CDC, 1998). As of December 1999, the number of women with AIDS in the United States had increased to 124,045 or 16.9 percent (CDC, 2000a).

The greatest increase in the number of AIDS cases has been among women of color. "Researchers estimate that 240,00-325,000 African Americans—about 1 in 50 African-American men and 1 in 160 African-American women—are infected with HIV. Of those infected with HIV, it is estimated that more than 106,000 African Americans are living with AIDS" (CDC, 2000c, p. 1). The CDC (1999a) reported for 1998 that 64,345 or 56.7 percent of AIDS cases among women were African-American. African-American women make up 57.3 percent (71,089) of AIDS cases among American women (CDC, 2000a), and 67.6 percent (23,131) of cases of HIV infection (CDC, 2000e). HIV/AIDS is the leading cause of death among African-American women ages twenty-five to forty-four (CDC, 2000d). African-American females currently represent 26.1 percent and 36.0 percent of all African Americans infected with AIDS and HIV, respectively (CDC, 2000a,e). In 2000, African-American women reported HIV transmission through injection drug use (IDU) or through heterosexual contact with an IDU, a bisexual male, a person with hemophilia, a transfusion recipient with HIV, or an HIV-infected person (CDC, 2000c).

Although Louisiana has experienced a 32 percent decline in the number of cases of new HIV infections since 1993, African Americans, who make up approximately 32 percent of the state's population, comprised 75 percent of the new cases of HIV reported in 1999. The rate of new infections for African Americans was 63/100,000—seven times that of whites and three times the rate for Hispanics. Sexually transmitted disease rates, which are likely to contribute to higher numbers of cases of HIV/AIDS, are also much higher for African Americans than other groups in Louisiana (Louisiana Department of Health and Hospitals [LDHH], 2001c). The Baton Rouge area ranks highest of Louisiana cities for AIDS case rates since 1999 and twelfth highest among U.S. cities. The Greater New Orleans area is ranked fourteenth in AIDS case rates among U.S. cities (LDHH, 2001c).

LOUISIANA AFRICAN-AMERICAN WOMEN

Historical Overview

The Atlantic slave trade brought 10 million slaves to America. After suffering physical pain, psychological despair, and mental anguish, the seasoned New World African Americans found that to survive they had to adjust to a new and alien environment. Slaves brought to Louisiana were from the African regions of Guinea, the Gold Coast, and Angola, and from the French islands of the Caribbean (Cummins, 1997). The cultural mores and values for these groups of slaves varied from region to region (Mills, 1977). Kein (1999) summarized the mixture of ethnic groups that make up the cultural landscape of Louisiana:

> An amazing variety of people from all over the world contributed to the making of the state of Louisiana—French, Spanish, German, Canadians, Acadians, Irish, Jewish, Chinese, Italians, Eastern Europeans, and a number of Indio Asians. . . . Africans, both slave and free and mixed people of the Caribbean and South America contributed their part. . . . Many of these people are lumped for commercial reasons under the ubiquitous and ambiguous labels of Cajun or Creole. (p. 119)

Because of historical confusion about these terms (Kein, 1999) and a current effort in the United States toward redefining race and ethnicity (Redefining race in America, 2000), for the purposes of this discussion, the following terms are defined to differentiate among Louisiana's groups:

- African American: an American of black African descent.
- Black: a person belonging to a dark-skinned race or one stemming in part from such a race, especially a Negro.
- Creole: a person of mixed French or Spanish and Negro descent speaking a dialect of French or Spanish.
- Free person of color ("gens de couleur libre"): persons of color not classified as slaves but neither afforded equal status with Europeans and their white descendants, many of whom could pass as white (Kein, 1999).
- Slave: a person held in servitude as the chattel of another.

In *Cane River,* the African-American author, Lalita Tademy (2001), reconstructs the story of her family, part African American, part white, some of whom were slaves and some slave owners. Susan Larson, book editor for the *Times Picayune* (2001, p. D-6), comments:

> Tademy brings home again and again the idea of what personal freedom means through showing what it is not—not speaking, not moving, not having any legal recourse for real injustice or oppression, not being able to have a wedding without the repeated admonition during the ceremony that a union of two slaves only exists at the whim of white masters. She shows us the fear and chaos that comes after a plantation owner's death, the cruel reality of a slave auction that divides families, even when slaves and buyers know each other personally. With the aid of family trees, she traces the complex history of an interracial family composed of slaves, free people of color, Creoles and white people. Tademy faces head-on realities of Black racism (the separation between gens de couleur libre and slaves, black mothers who hope that their daughters can gain the attention and protection of white men). (Susan Larson [2001], Memory Banks, from the April 15, 2003, issue of *The Times-Picayune* © 2003 The Times-Picayune Publishing Co. All rights reserved. Used with permission of *The Times-Picayune.*)

Southern cultural transformation was rapid as slave owners established measures to reward those slaves who learned English, acquired new skills, and embraced Christianity. "Those who readily accepted new values, called 'New Negroes,' and those born on American soil, called 'Creoles', could expect preferential treatment, special privileges, and more prestigious jobs" (Schweninger, 1989, p. 193). Creoles of color participated politically and economically, were educated, and even participated in philanthropy (Kein, 1999). Free people of color were not classified as slaves but neither were they able to enjoy equal status with the Europeans and their white descendants. Kein (1999) refers to this group as "gens de couleur libre" and points out that many were able to pass as white enjoying the advantages of such status.

Slaves lived on plantations, in cities, and towns. Upon discarding the manners and attitudes of field hands, their social situations improved. Those slaves who assimilated into the dominant culture moved into what was known as "quasi freedom"—halfway between bondage and freedom. Once in the city, they lived independent, autonomous lives, securing their own employment, maintaining their own families, and were able to move about from place to place (Schweninger, 1989). Farm and plantation slaves in Louisiana, on the other hand, developed cultural mores and attitudes peculiar to their unique circumstances. Folktales and folk beliefs were used through kinship networks to transmit social values and attitudes from parents to children and from shamans to other slaves (Schweninger, 1989). Social values and attitudes were and continue to be as diverse as the cultural and ethnic groups that make up Louisiana's people (Kein, 1999).

Tademy (2001), Mills (1977), and many others have written narratives and other accounts of life in Louisiana among slaves, free people of color, Creoles, and other mixed races of people. Wallace (1978) points out that two archetypes of the African-American female emerged from slavery: the Black Lady—the privileged woman who had either been free before the war or maintained a special position in a white household, sometimes as the mistress of a white master; and the Amazon—the breeder who was bigger, stronger, tougher, more rebellious, and usually poor. By the 1950s, the upper class of African-American society tended to rate beauty and merit on the basis of the lightness of the skin, the straightness of hair, and other features, creating a community plagued by color discrimination. White features bore a more reliable ticket into this society than professional status or higher education (Wallace, 1978). Harris (1995) highlights the issue of colorism relative to skin tone. She defines it as the prejudicial or preferential treatment of same-race people based on their color, and the ascribed value and privilege given to a same-race person based on lightness of color. "Underdeveloping the pictures of dark-skinned people in my college yearbook so no one looked too dark was colorism" (Harris, 1995, p. 75). As a dark-skinned person, she referred to the pain of colorism within her family as the experience of a prison of color that fostered self-hatred, anger, invisibility, inadequacy, and over/underachieving. Historical attitudes toward skin color and this phenomenon of colorism have fostered racism within a race by discrimination of light-skinned African Americans against dark-skinned African Americans.

Current Status

Today, African-American women in Louisiana come in all skin complexions, from very fair to almost blue-black. The history of Louisiana, with its cultural and ethnic diversity, unmatched by any other region in the United States, established a backdrop that accounts for this uniqueness. When compared to other women in the United States, Louisiana women differ not only on ethnic and cultural factors, but also on several demographic variables. African-American women make up one-third of Louisiana women compared to 13 percent of women in the rest of the nation. Louisiana women are younger, fewer live in metropolitan areas, and are more likely to be the head of their families than women in other states. According to the IWPR (1998),

> women in Louisiana are less likely than women nationally to graduate from high school and have full-time, year-round employment. Those who are employed earn considerably less than women in other states (and Louisiana men) and they are less likely to have health insurance. What Louisiana women experience more of is poverty. (p. 1)

Louisiana women face serious obstacles in attaining standing comparable to the average for women in the United States. Two composite indices utilized by the IWPR rank all Louisiana women forty-seventh out of the fifty states and the District of Columbia in employment and economic autonomy. Louisiana women also rank low in standard of living, are worse off than men, and lack rights crucial to achieving equality with men (IWPR, 1998). Louisiana women earn much lower wages than women in the nation as a whole do even though more than 62 percent with children under age eighteen are working. Twenty-one percent of Louisiana women live in poverty, and 19 percent lack health insurance and the basic necessities of life (IWPR, 1998).

HIV/AIDS is endemic among the poor and disadvantaged people of Louisiana, especially among African-American women. Since 1993, a consistent increase has occurred in the proportion of HIV/AIDS cases among Louisiana females. In 1993, females accounted for only 21 percent of new infections (LDHH, 2001c). By 1999, 30 percent of all new HIV infections were among women, 85 percent of whom were African American. The year-end data for 1998 report 10,180 adult cases of AIDS, including 1,355 women. The 1990 AIDS case rates reveal a rate of 6.1/100,000 for African-American females. By 1996, the rate had increased fivefold to 30.6/100,000 for that same group (LDHH, 1999). In contrast, the rates for white females were 1.4/100,000 in 1990 and 2.3/100,000 in 1996. "Recently the African-American female case rate [in Louisiana] surpassed that of white males" (LDHH, 1999, p. 34).

The surveillance data released by LDHH on February 28, 2001, reported 549 cases of AIDS and 1,568 cases of HIV infection among living adult and adolescent females. African-American females constituted 80 and 84 percent of those same groups, respectively. Heterosexual contact was reported among females as the mode of transmission for 36.4 percent of all AIDS cases. Although only 51.5 percent of adult females with HIV infection reported a mode of transmission for infection, 60.5 percent of those that did reported being infected through heterosexual contact (LDHH, 2001a, 2001b).

The LDHH HIV/AIDS Prevention Plan for 1999 through 2001 targeted females at risk for heterosexual transmission as primarily African-American, noninjection drug users, injection drug users, partners of injection drug users and bisexual men. The CDC recommends that the components for Louisiana's Comprehensive HIV Prevention Program include objectives for target populations and interventions. The prevention interventions for racial/ethnic minorities and sexually active females incorporate venue-based outreach; condom availability; street outreach; popular opinion leader; HIV counseling, testing, and referral; partner counseling and referral services; and peer-led small group sessions. The efficacy of these interventions, as determined through national prevention intervention programs and their evaluation, are viewed through a Euro-American epistemology rather than one that encompasses historical, cultural, and regional differences.

ETHNIC EPISTEMOLOGY

The Euro-American epistemological tradition and the African epistemological tradition represent two distinct and divergent perspectives. The Euro-American perspective rests on the premise that the individual mind is the source of knowledge and existence. In contrast, the African epistemology asserts that the individual's existence and knowledge is contingent upon relationships with others (Ladson-Billings, 2000).

DuBois (1903/1989) wrote, "One ever feels his twoness—an American, a Negro; two souls, two thoughts, two unreconciled strivings; two warring ideals in one dark body." (p. 3). He and other scholars (Gilroy, 1993; Norton 1993) have developed epistemological stances informed by their own culture and identity. Multiple consciousness (double consciousness/dual perspective) is a transcendent position allowing one to see and understand positions of inclusion and exclusion—margin and mainstream (Ladson-Billings, 2000). In present-day social work, the dual perspective is utilized in several models that serve to understand diversity and to focus on differences in human behavior (Tanner, 1992; Norton, 1993).

Ladson-Billings (2000) discusses the idea that racialized labels unite groups for political and cultural purposes. These labels serve as groupings to acknowledge some common experiences as group members. She also discusses the fact that others argue in favor of a perspective advantage as the constructed other in instances when a dual perspective has emerged among groups. This position contends a belief that the poor and working classes have a perspective of their own experiences while simultaneously grasping the fundamentals of the workings of the dominant class.

> Thus the work of this liminal perspective is to reveal the ways that dominant perspectives distort the realities of the other in an effort to maintain power relations that continue to disadvantage those who are locked out of the mainstream. (Ladson-Billings, 2000, p. 263)

What constitutes reality in the minority culture thus takes on the character of deviant behavior by the dominant culture.

Wallace (1978) illuminated the myths of the black macho male and the black superwoman and illustrated the impact of the two epistemologies as they translated into African-American culture. She discussed the existence of the pressure generated by the dominant white standard and the existence of an African standard laid down by slaves. African cultural mores provided for trial marriage, pregnancy followed by marriage, and for some degree of sexual experimentation prior to settling down. Once the African slave trade was discontinued, female slaves of childbearing age were used as the source for children to satisfy the labor demands of a swelling colonial population (Mills, 1977), thus reinforcing African cultural norms. The emancipation of slaves demanded assimilation into and adaptation of the social norms and mores of the dominant culture. It was only after blacks accepted Euro-American standards for family life, manhood, and womanhood that black men and women began to resent one another, thus creating discord within their families and culture (Wallace, 1978). These behavioral rules, forcibly or otherwise, are the very behaviors that currently put African-American women in Louisiana at immense vulnerability for HIV infection transmitted via heterosexual contact as is reflected statistically.

The Euro-American epistemology and its perspectives define African Americans (blacks) as a homogenous group. However, the cultural and ethnic differences resonant in Louisiana's population of mixed groups constitute values, norms, and mores uniquely different from other parts of the United States. Heterogeneity within the race and the preferential treatment given to those of mixed race and lighter skin complexion served to create an atmosphere of racism among southern African Americans as prevalent as that against the African-American population as a whole. An ethnic epistemological perspective substantiates the feasibility of theoretical stances that acknowledge the inclusion of a double-consciousness approach to research with cultural groups different from the dominant culture.

CULTURE IN PREVENTION EFFORTS

Researchers have determined numerous cultural and social factors associated with the sexual behaviors of African-American women that put them at risk for HIV infection (Choi and Catania, 1996; Kusseling et al., 1996; O'Sullivan and Gaines, 1998; Pete and DeSantis, 1990; Sobo, 1993; Wingood and DiClemente, 1996). Gagnon and Simon (1973) introduced the notion of sexual scripts. They viewed all people as actors with parts in scripts that exist for sexual life. Laws and Schwartz (1977) wrote that the socialization of children occurs in the family and is primarily controlled by the parents who control what reality children are exposed to and what conceptual tools they have for problem solving. They further wrote that the first component of sexual identity rests upon sex-role categories, which constitute a basic division in society.

Sexual identity evolves as the individual attempts to match her own experience with the available sexual scripts. She learns the language that is applied to sexual feelings and events, as well as society's expectations for a person of her age and sex (Laws and Schwartz, 1977).

Allgeier and McCormick (1983) described the second sexual response system as the psychosocial system, based on the culture's sexual scripts for appropriate male and female behavior.

The diversity of the Louisiana "Gumbo" cultural landscape and its ethnic nuances qualitatively provides for the suitable application of the dual perspective in intrastate scientific research. However, research efforts in HIV/AIDS prevention have applied theories to African Americans as a homogenous group that lack adequate cultural modifications for their effectiveness among Louisiana's African-American females. Examination of cultural aspects within Louisiana's borders may reveal factors that hinder the effectiveness of HIV prevention interventions utilized in the South thus far. The application of qualitative research methodology may provide a more appropriate venue to capture the caveats of cognitive reasoning and sexual behaviors of Louisiana's African-American females that may differ from other U.S. African-American women.

Heightening professional awareness among social workers on the more intimate factors relative to the sexual behaviors of African-American women in Louisiana would substantially contribute to a knowledge base required to stop the spread of HIV. However, any new insights qualitatively determined will provide for assimilation into the design and implementation of HIV/AIDS prevention interventions within ethnically diverse communities. Social workers engaged in providing services to African-American female populations may creatively interweave HIV prevention interventions into their initiatives to empower women with attitudes and skills that could contribute to better decisions regarding sexual intimacy in the face of devastating HIV/AIDS statistics.

Bing et al. (1990) stated:

> AIDS is no different from other illnesses that are endemic among the poor and disadvantaged people of our society. No other condition, however, arouses so much social and racial

prejudice, adding discrimination and ill will to the sufferings of persons with AIDS. (p. 69)

It is with immense consequence that AIDS continues to spread and disproportionately impact the African-American women of this country and more specifically in Louisiana. The numbers are large enough without statistical privilege to the full spectrum of the epidemic among African-American women in Louisiana. That would be even more disheartening.

REFERENCES

Allgeier, E. R. and McCormick, N. B. (1983). *Changing boundaries: Gender roles and sexual behavior.* Palo Alto, CA: Mayfield Publishing.

Bing, E. G., Nichols, S. E., Goldfinger, S. M., Fernandez, F., Cabaj, R., Dodley, R. G., Jr., Krener, P., Prager, M., and Ruiz, P. (1990). The many faces of AIDS: Opportunities for intervention. *New Directions for Mental Health Services, 48,* 69-81.

Centers for Disease Control and Prevention (1995). Update: AIDS among women—United States, 1994. *Morbidity and Mortality Weekly Report, 44*(5), 81-84.

Centers for Disease Control and Prevention (1996). Update: Mortality attributable to HIV infection among persons aged 25-44 years—United States, 1994. *Morbidity and Mortality Weekly Report, 45,* 121-125.

Centers for Disease Control and Prevention (1998). AIDS cases by sex, age at diagnosis, and race/ethnicity, reported through December 1997, United States. *HIV/AIDS Surveillance Report, 9*(2), 16.

Centers for Disease Control and Prevention (1999a). AIDS cases by sex, age at diagnosis, and race/ethnicity, reported through December 1998. *HIV/AIDS Surveillance Report, 10*(2), Table 7.

Centers for Disease Control and Prevention (1999b). HIV infection cases by sex, age at diagnosis, and race/ethnicity, reported through December 1998, from the 33 areas with confidential HIV infection reporting. *HIV/AIDS Surveillance Report, 10*(2), Table 8.

Centers for Disease Control and Prevention (2000a). AIDS cases by sex, age at diagnosis, and race/ethnicity, reported through December, 1999, United States. *HIV/AIDS Surveillance Report, 11*(2), Table 7.

Centers for Disease Control and Prevention (2000b). AIDS cases in racial and ethnic minorities, January 1986-June 1998, United States. HIV/AIDS Surveillance Report by race/ethnicity: Slide #1-8. Available online at <http://www.cdc.gov/nchstp/hiv_aids/graphics/images/1238/1238-1.htm>.

Centers for Disease Control and Prevention (2000c). Fact Sheet—HIV/AIDS among African Americans. NCHSTP-Division of HIV/AIDS prevention. *HIV/*

AIDS among African Americans. Available online at <http://www.cdc.gov/nchstp/hiv_aids/pubs/ facts/afam.htm>.

Centers for Disease Control and Prevention (2000d). Fact Sheet—HIV/AIDS among US women. *HIV/AIDS Among US Women: Minority and Young Women at Continuing Risk.* Available online at <http://www.cdc.gov/nchstp/hiv_aids/pubs/facts/women.htm>.

Centers for Disease Control and Prevention (2000e). HIV infection cases by sex, age at diagnosis, and race/ethnicity, reported through December, 1999, from the 34 areas with confidential HIV infection reporting. *HIV/AIDS Surveillance Report, 11*(2), Table 8.

Centers for Disease Control and Prevention (2000f). Persons reported to be living with HIV infection and with AIDS, by state and age group, reported through December 1999. *HIV/AIDS Surveillance Report, 11*(2), Table 1.

Choi, K. H. and Catania, J. A. (1996). Changes in multiple sex partnerships, HIV testing, and condom use among U.S. heterosexuals 18-49 years of age. *American Journal of Public Health, 86,* 554-556.

Cummins, L. T. (1997). Louisiana as a French colony. In B. H. Wall (Ed.), *Louisiana: A history* (pp. 21-39). Wheeling, IL: Harlan Davidson, Inc.

Du Bois, W. E. B. (1903/1989). *The souls of black folk.* New York: Bantam Books.

Dunn, J. L. (1998). Defining women. *Journal of Contemporary Ethnography, 26*(4), 479-510.

Fields, C. (1992). Women and AIDS: Mother and child relationship. *FAS and other drugs update, 11*(2), 1.

Gagnon, J. and Simon, W. (1973). *Sexual conduct: The social sources of human sexuality.* Chicago: Aldine.

Gilroy, P. (1993). *The black Atlantic.* Cambridge, MA: Harvard University Press.

Harris, V. R. (1995). Prison of color. In J. Adleman and G. M. Enguidanos (Eds.), *Racism in the lives of women* (pp. 75-83). Binghamton, NY: The Haworth Press.

Henderson, G. J. (Ed.). (1993). *The United States government manual 1993/94.* Washington, DC: U. S. Government Printing Office.

Institute for Women's Policy Research (1998). The status of women in Louisiana. Washington, DC: Author.

James, T. (Speaker) (1994). Regional AIDS interfaith network, National Skills Building Conference (Cassette recording No. 413). Washington, DC: National Minority AIDS Council.

Kein, S. (1999). *Gumbo people* (Revised edition). New Orleans, LA: Margaret Media.

Kusseling, F. S., Shapiro, M. F., Greenberg, J. M., and Wenger, N. S. (1996). Understanding why heterosexual adults do not practice safer sex: A comparison of two samples. *AIDS Education and Prevention, 8*(3), 247-257.

Ladson-Billings, G. (2000). Racialized discourses and ethnic epistemologies. In N. K. Denzin and Y. S. Lincoln (Eds.), *Handbook of qualitative research* (pp. 257-277). Thousand Oaks, CA: Sage.

Land, H. (1994). AIDS and women of color. *Families in Society,* June, 355-361.

Larson, S. (2001). Memory banks. *The Times Picayune,* April 15, p. D-6.

Laws, J. L. and Schwartz, P. (1977). *Sexual scripts: The social construction of female sexuality.* Hinsdale, IL: The Dryden Press.

Louisiana Department of Health and Hospitals (1999). Statewide plan. *Louisiana HIV/AIDS statewide prevention plan* (pp. 28-46). New Orleans: Author.

Louisiana Department of Health and Hospitals (2000). Statewide plan. *Louisiana HIV/AIDS statewide prevention plan* (pp. 32-53). New Orleans: Author.

Louisiana Department of Health and Hospitals (2001a). Acquired immunodeficiency syndrome, prevalent AIDS cases in Louisiana. *Surveillance Report,* February 28, 1.

Louisiana Department of Health and Hospitals (2001b). Prevalence of HIV infected persons in Louisiana. *Surveillance Report,* February 28, 1.

Louisiana Department of Health and Hospitals (2001c). Statewide plan. *Louisiana HIV/AIDS Statewide Prevention Plan,* Part 1, 1-29.

Mills, G. B. (1977). *The forgotten people.* Baton Rouge, LA: Louisiana State University Press.

National Pediatric HIV Resource Center (1992). *Children, adolescents, women and families with AIDS* (Flyer). Washington, DC: Author.

Norton, D. G. (1993). Diversity, early socialization, and temporal development: The dual perspective revisited. *Social Work, 38*(1), 82-90.

O'Sullivan, L. F. and Gaines, M. E. (1998). Decision making in college students' heterosexual dating relationships: Ambivalence about engaging in sexual activity. *Journal of Social and Personal Relationships, 15*(3), 347-363.

Pete, J. M. and DeSantis, L. (1990). Sexual decision making in young black adolescent females. *Adolescence, 25*(97), 145-154.

Redefining race in America [special report] (2000). *Newsweek,* September 18, pp. 38-65.

Satcher, D. (Speaker). (1994). Welcome and opening remarks, National Skills Building Conference (Cassette Recording No. 100). Washington, DC: National Minority AIDS Council.

Schweninger, L. (1989). Slave culture. In C. R. Wilson and W. Ferris (Eds.), *Encyclopedia of southern culture* (pp. 192-193). Chapel Hill, NC: The University of North Carolina Press.

Sobo, E. J. (1993). Inner-city women and AIDS: The psychosocial benefit of unsafe sex. *Culture, Medicine and Psychiatry, 17,* 455-485.

Tademy, L. (2001). *Cane river.* New York: Warner Books.

Tanner, Z. (1992). School counselors and at-risk adolescents: Integrating family and subcultural perspectives. *Family Therapy, 19*(1), 33-42.

Wallace, M. (1978). *Black macho and the myth of the super-woman.* New York: Warner Books.

Wingood, G. M. and DiClemente, R. J. (1996). HIV sex risk reduction interventions for women: A review. *American Journal of Preventive Medicine, 12,* 209-217.

Index

Page numbers followed by the letter "f" indicate figures; those followed by the letter "t" indicate tables.

T - #0522 - 101024 - C0 - 212/152/13 - PB - 9780789023025 - Gloss Lamination